5-INGREDIENT
ALKALINE DIET
COOKBOOK

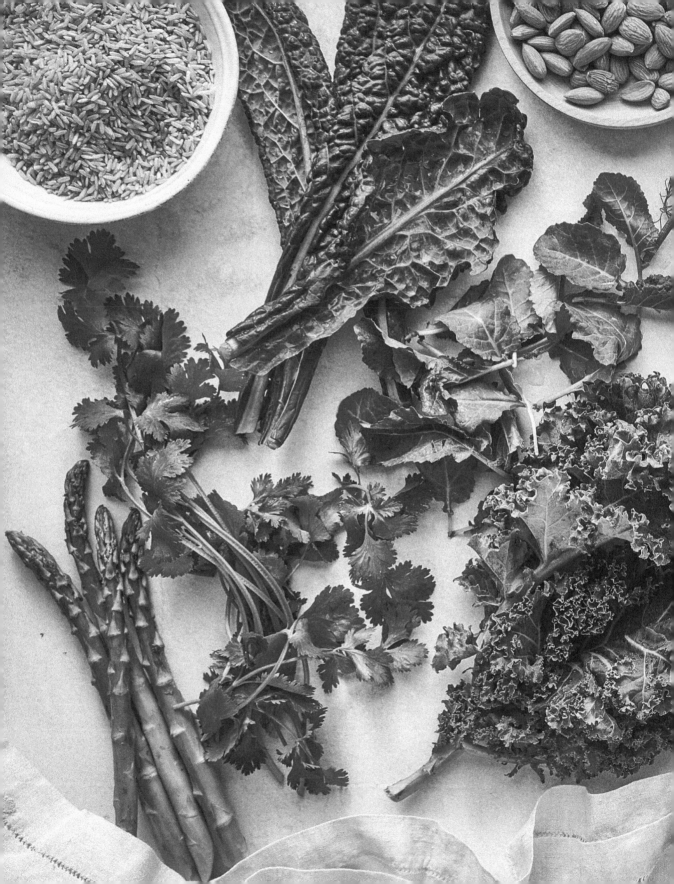

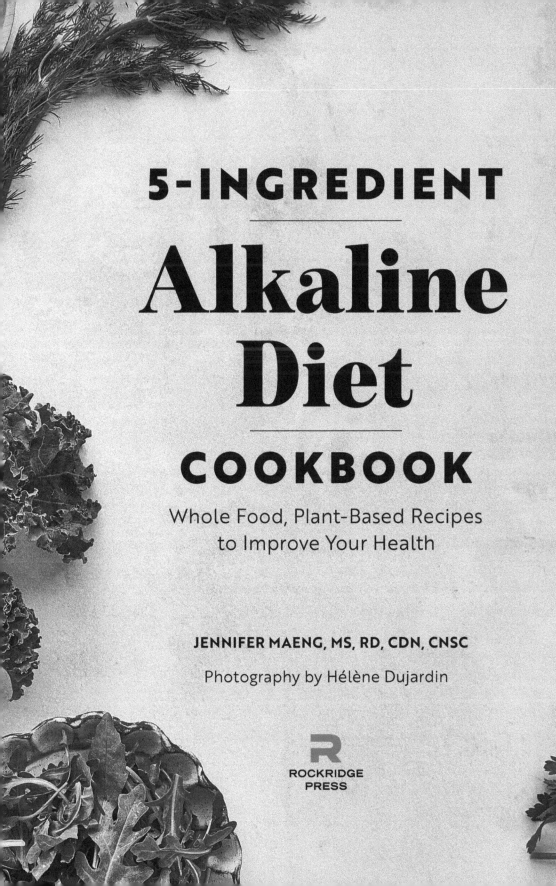

5-INGREDIENT

Alkaline Diet

COOKBOOK

Whole Food, Plant-Based Recipes
to Improve Your Health

JENNIFER MAENG, MS, RD, CDN, CNSC

Photography by Hélène Dujardin

ROCKRIDGE
PRESS

For general information on our other products and services or to obtain technical support, please contact our Customer Care Department within the United States at (866) 744-2665, or outside the United States at (510) 253-0500.

Rockridge Press publishes its books in a variety of electronic and print formats. Some content that appears in print may not be available in electronic books, and vice versa.

Interior and Cover Designer: Elizabeth Zuhl
Art Producer: Sara Feinstein
Editor: Annie Choi
Production Manager: Riley Hoffman

Photography © 2021 Hélène Dujardin. Food styling by Anna Hampton.
Author photo courtesy of Rebecca Enis.

Paperback ISBN: 978-1-64739-960-3 | eBook ISBN: 978-1-64739-961-0
R0

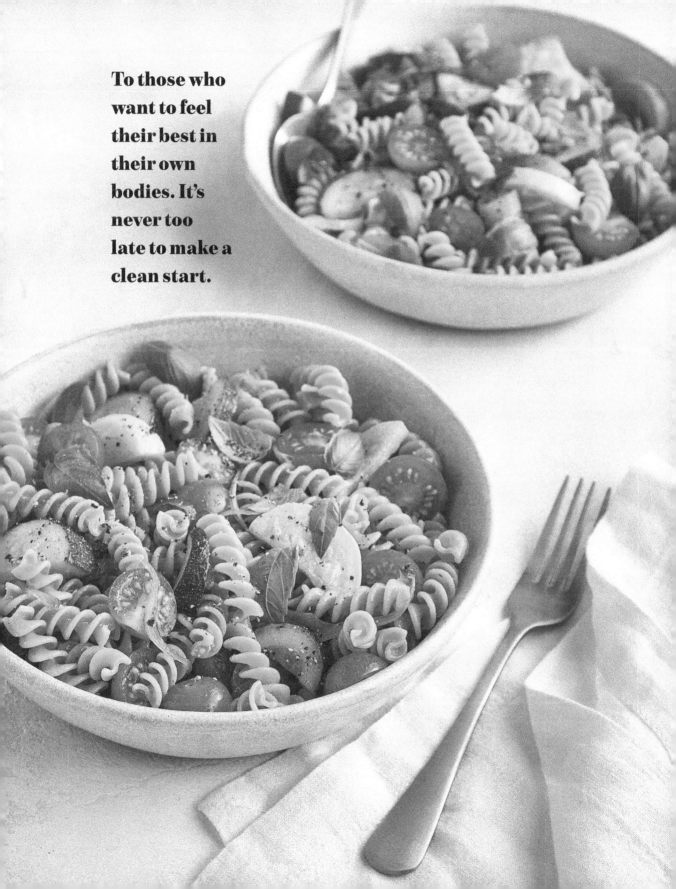

To those who want to feel their best in their own bodies. It's never too late to make a clean start.

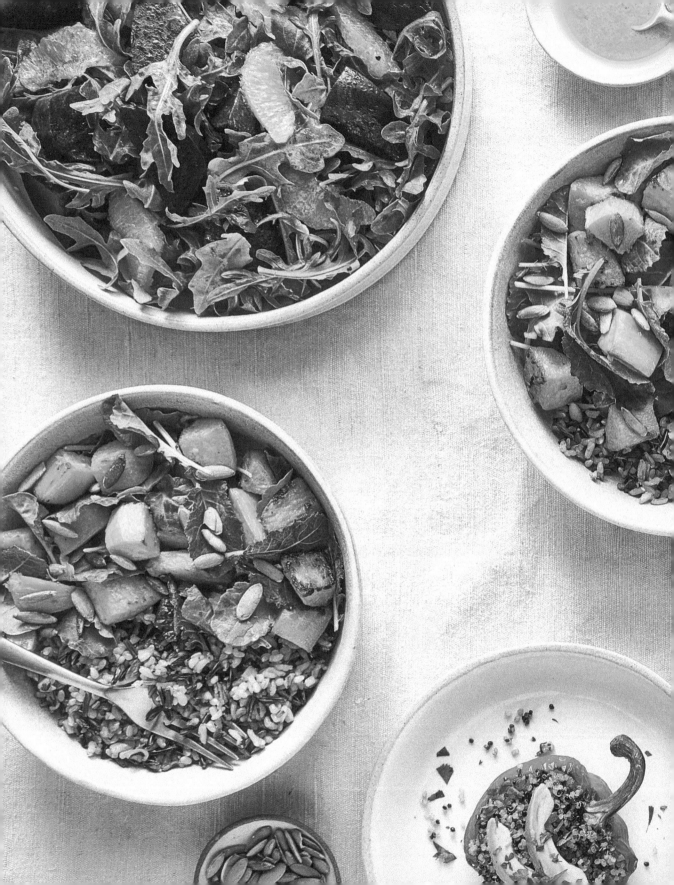

Contents

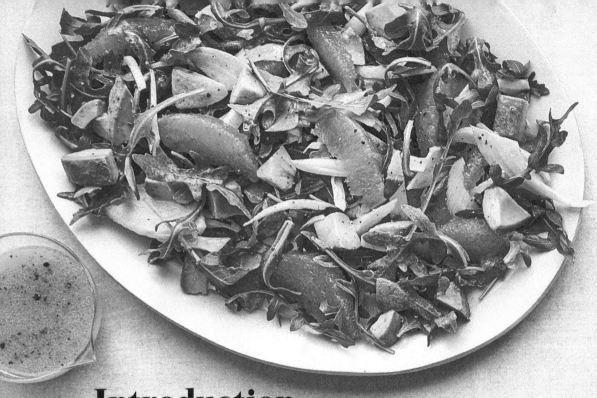

Introduction

Last summer, I had my second child. As joyful as I was, I realized that I needed to prioritize my health more than ever to keep up with my growing nutrition counseling practice and caring for my family. So I transitioned to a more plant-based diet consisting mainly of vegetables, fruits, nuts, seeds, plant-based oils, whole grains, and beans—all hallmarks of the alkaline diet.

This mostly plant-based diet not only helped me lose my baby weight but also helped reduce inflammation from postpartum stress and many sleepless nights. I had more energy throughout the day and was no longer relying on coffee for energy. And because I had gestational diabetes during both of my pregnancies, eating more plant-based meals was important to minimize insulin spikes to prevent chronic disease.

The rates of disease linked to obesity and lifestyle are higher than ever. In America, 19 percent of children and 42 percent of adults are not just overweight but obese, putting them at risk for diabetes, stroke, heart disease, and cancer. As a reaction to this growing health crisis, new diets pop up every year, along with new lines of processed foods to accommodate those diets.

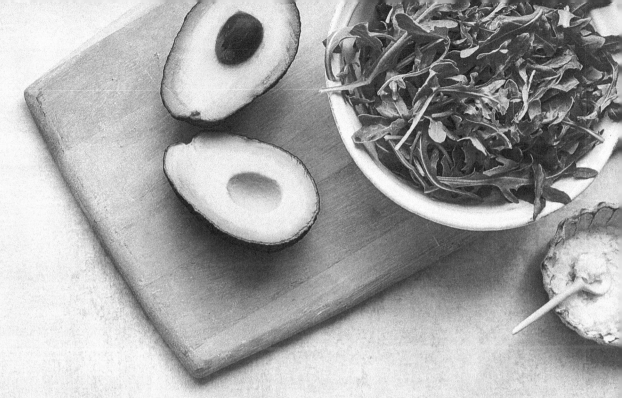

You've probably heard of the alkaline diet from friends, online articles, or even celebrities devoted to eating this way. In its essence, the alkaline diet is a plant-based diet that focuses on nutrient-dense whole foods to bring balance to your body. It allows the body to function at its best by reducing inflammation and thereby increasing the body's ability to fight disease.

Our bodies are highly capable of maintaining homeostasis, but a consistently poor diet made up of processed foods interferes with our body's ability to remain in balance. When this happens, the body will use all of its resources to make sure our bodily systems can function as they should. Every time our bodies have to fight imbalances, we are harming every system, including hormone function, the immune system, the digestive system, and the body's capacity to detox and maintain its pH balance. The alkaline diet can improve your health and reduce this unnecessary burden on your body. (We'll get into the evidence-based reasons the alkaline diet can be so healthy—and not all of them are related to pH.)

Cooking and eating fresh, wholesome foods doesn't have to be a chore, either. In this book I'll show you how you can use the alkaline diet to introduce more whole-food, plant-based meals into your lifestyle with 90 simple recipes—all using just five ingredients or less. It doesn't get much easier.

Let's get started!

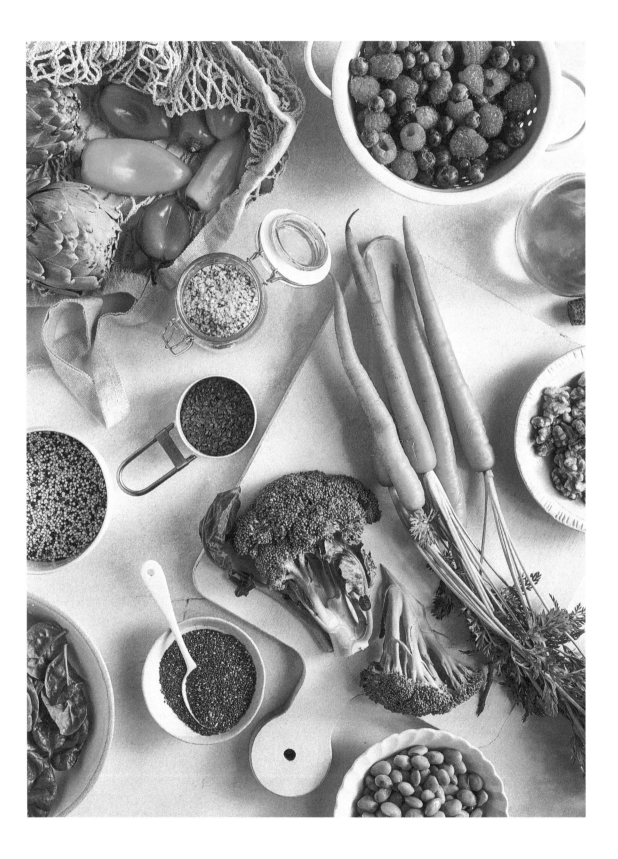

CHAPTER ONE

What Is the Alkaline Diet?

• • • • •

Interest in the alkaline diet has grown around the world. According to *U.S. News & World Report*, the alkaline diet was one of the top 10 most searched-for diets in 2020, along with the Whole30 and Paleo diets, which share similar protocols. In this chapter, I will lay out what the alkaline diet is and how you can follow it. I will also explain the mechanisms behind the alkaline diet, such as homeostasis, and even debunk common alkaline diet myths so you can best use the diet for your health.

The Alkaline Diet Made Simple

The alkaline diet consists of whole, plant-based foods and focuses on specific foods that are believed to be alkaline-producing in the body. It is based on the idea that eating acid-forming foods can cause metabolic imbalance, which in turn can lead to chronic disease. Although there is no scientific evidence to date for the pH-related benefits of the alkaline diet, it is undoubtedly a nutritious diet because it focuses on eating wholesome, nutrient-dense foods.

Whenever I introduce a new dietary regimen to my clients, I tell them to try to follow it most of the time. A most-of-the-time approach is typically more successful than a more rigid approach, which often leads to failure and disappointment. For the alkaline diet, I suggest an 80/20 approach, in which 80 percent of the foods you eat are alkaline foods (think vegan) and 20 percent are acidic foods. This 20 percent is not necessarily reserved for beers, burgers, and fries; it should consist of acidic foods that are still nutritious—such as fish, eggs, and whole grains—but acidic. All the recipes in this book are alkaline, which means all of them count toward the 80 percent of your meals.

All foods have their own pH and their own effect on your body's pH. Animal-based foods can have acidifying effects in your body, yet plant-based foods such as fruits and vegetables have alkaline effects. It's important to note that the pH of a food does not determine its acid or alkaline effects. For example, lemon is acidic in its natural state, but when it is metabolized in your stomach, it becomes alkaline.

When your diet is mostly acidic foods, it can lead to inflammation. Studies have shown a positive association between a plant-based diet and reduced inflammation. Plant-based foods can promote healthy gut bacteria, can reduce inflammation, and have been associated with a lower body mass index (BMI), a measure of overall body fat based on height and weight. Similar to a vegan diet, the alkaline diet focuses on eating mostly plant-based foods to maximize nutrient intake and minimize inflammation for optimal health.

The Alkaline Diet in Five Ingredients

My motivation in writing this book is to show you how amazing you can feel when your diet consists of whole, fresh, natural ingredients. According to a study published in the journal *Public Health Nutrition*, we are more likely to eat less sugar, and less likely to overeat, when we cook most of our meals at home. But many people think of the kitchen as a place to work and not a place for comfort, joy, and nourishment. As a registered dietitian, I help clients gain more confidence in the kitchen and enjoy their time cooking by sharing simple recipes that they'll be excited to try.

The simple five-ingredient approach of this book is designed to help you learn how to eat healthfully with minimal stress. It will also make it easier to develop an intuitive understanding of what a mostly alkaline diet should look like, because you'll see similar ingredients used in different ways.

And of course, food needs to be delicious—not only for enjoyment but also so that the flavorful results will bring you back to the kitchen again and again, making you more likely to reach your dietary goals. With the five-ingredient approach, you'll see that making nutritious, healthy, delicious meals doesn't need to be complicated.

The Science of pH

The human body is around 70 percent water, and that water can have either acidic or alkaline properties. The scale that measures acidity levels is called the pH (potential hydrogen) scale. pH levels range from 1 to 6.9 (acidic) and 7.1 to 14 (alkaline), with 7 being neutral.

Different parts of our bodies need different degrees of acidity or alkalinity to carry out their diverse functions. For example, the pH in saliva ranges from 6.5 to 7.5. In the stomach, pH can be as low as 1 when foods are being digested, but when they leave the stomach, their pH rises to around 4. And pH levels can range from 4 to 7 in the trip from the small intestine to the large intestine, depending on the digestive process being carried out.

The ideal pH of blood is 7.4—slightly alkaline. Unlike the digestive system, the body regulates the pH of blood to remain alkaline at between 7.36 to 7.44, regardless of what you eat. A pH in this specific range is necessary for optimal physical functioning, so our bodies use various ways to regulate blood pH.

Scientists have used different methods to analyze the acidity and alkalinity of food. For the alkaline diet, ideal foods are measured using the potential renal acid load (PRAL) method. Developed by researchers Thomas Remer and Friedrich Manz, PRAL scores show the amount of acid load left in your body after food has been digested (known as metabolic waste). In general, animal-based proteins, such as meat, cheese, and eggs, increase the production of acid in your body, and fruits and vegetables increase alkalinity.

However, there is no scientific evidence that the acidity or alkalinity of the metabolic waste left behind after food is digested changes the pH of your blood. Maintaining proper blood pH in the body *is* important, since high acidity levels can lead to disease and the growth of harmful bacteria, which thrive in a highly acidic environment. But maintaining blood pH is an automatically regulated process. In other words, the body does it on its own, regardless of what you eat. So why is diet important in this process?

To return to normal pH levels, the body must obtain minerals from organs, bones, and tissue in an attempt to neutralize the acidity. This process can, over time, weaken the body, demineralize the bones, and cause various health problems. So although overindulging in acid-forming foods may not directly change your blood pH, it can overwork your body in its efforts to maintain homeostasis, which may affect inflammation and kidney health.

Although the foods you eat cannot change your blood pH, they can have an impact on your saliva and urine pH. One of the ways your body regulates blood pH is by excretion through the urine. When you eat a steak, for example, your urine will be acidic as your body tries to remove the metabolic waste of that acidic food. When you eat vegetables, your urine tends to be more alkaline.

Why the Alkaline Diet Is So Good for You

Followers of the alkaline diet believe that you can alkalize the body and improve health by eating alkaline foods and avoiding foods that leave an

SHOULD YOU TEST YOUR PH?

Some people who follow the alkaline diet will test their urine or saliva pH with at-home test strips. As I've explained, testing your saliva or urine pH does not reflect the pH of your blood. Saliva pH can also vary widely depending on factors such as dental hygiene and the flora that lives in your mouth. The pH of your urine can be affected by your kidney function and the types and amount of food you eat. For example, if you happen to eat an acidic food such as bagels on a particular day, the pH of your urine will likely be acidic, but this may not be helpful in understanding your blood pH.

That said, if you are curious and want to check your saliva or urine pH, here's how.

- **Saliva pH strip:** To test the pH of your saliva, fill your mouth with saliva, and spit. Fill your mouth again with saliva and place a small amount of it on your pH strip. A number higher than 7 indicates alkaline, and a number less than 7 indicates acid.

- **Urine pH strip:** Dip your test strip into your urine sample and match the result with the corresponding color and number that came with the test strip.

Ultimately, you should listen to your body as you try out different foods and monitor their effects. Rest assured that the types of foods you'll be eating on the alkaline diet can promote good health, whether or not you decide to test your pH levels.

ash residue (the end product of metabolism) in the body. This is known as the "acid-ash hypothesis," which states that foods like dairy, red meat, processed meat, alcohol, and sugars leave acid-ash residue in the body and retain a pH of 0 to 6 in the blood. Vegetables, whole grains, legumes, and fruits are considered alkaline and retain a pH of 8 to 14 in the blood. There are different versions of the alkaline diet, and some limit specific fruits, vegetables, and legumes.

Eating an alkaline-based diet is good for your health, but not in the ways many people are led to believe. The ash residue that is a byproduct of metabolism does not, in fact, affect the pH balance in the blood. Under most conditions, the body maintains a neutral pH of 7.35 to 7.45. Specific extreme conditions, such as diabetic ketoacidosis and some types of lung disease, can change the body's pH, but those instances require hospitalization.

However, current research shows that following a diet high in vegetables, fruit, whole grains, and legumes (while limiting added sugars, processed foods, red meat, and processed meat) decreases the risk of a variety of health conditions. An alkaline diet relies heavily on plant-based foods, which have been shown to be beneficial for overall health.

Here are common health conditions that can be improved by the alkaline diet, although perhaps not in the way you might expect.

Cancer

Cancer occurs when abnormal cells divide in a way that's out of control and destroy healthy body tissue. Proponents of the alkaline diet suggest that following the typical Western diet, which is abundant in processed foods, sugar, and animal proteins, can alter acid-base homeostasis in our bodies by creating an acidic environment and possibly helping cancer cells grow.

What We Know: Research conducted in animal and in vitro studies suggests that oral bicarbonates that make your urine or blood less acidic could be useful in treating cancer. However, there have been no credible studies on humans that show a correlation between pH and cancer.

The Bottom Line: According to the American Institute for Cancer Research, the World Cancer Research Fund International, and the American Cancer Society, eating red meat and processed meat, considered acid-forming in the alkaline diet, is associated with an increased risk of cancer. Researchers believe that the association between cancer and the consumption of red and processed meats is due to the saturated fat content, heme iron (a form of iron in animal foods that contains hemoglobin), and mutagens (any agent that causes genetic mutations) in these foods, not their pH level.

Research from these organizations also concluded that eating sugary foods and processed grains do not directly cause cancer or increase the body's acidity. However, the increased calories and lack of fiber from these foods lead to being overweight or obesity, which increases the risk of a variety of health conditions, including cancer, diabetes, and cardiovascular disease.

In short, it is the nutritional content of the alkaline foods that helps prevent cancer, not the pH.

Bone Health

Our bones are mostly made up of collagen fibers and minerals, and our bodies constantly break down and rebuild them. Bone health is determined by many different factors, including diet, medication, activity level, hormones, age, and alcohol use. The proponents of the alkaline diet believe that an acidic diet can lead to poor bone health.

What We Know: Supporters of the alkaline diet claim that eating alkaline foods reduces the chance of developing osteoporosis and that consuming acidic foods breaks down bone mass by making our bodies work harder to neutralize pH. When the body is low in minerals that come from alkalizing foods, minerals must come from the bones.

The Bottom Line: Studies have shown positive effects of an alkaline-focused diet on bone and muscle retention. Muscle retention is also important here, because poor muscle tone can also lead to increased risk of bone fracture, especially in elderly people.

Acid Reflux

Acid reflux is the heartburn and indigestion that occurs when stomach acids flow up the esophagus. Proponents of the alkaline diet believe that by eliminating foods that are acidic, heartburn and indigestion can be prevented.

What We Know: Those with gastroesophageal reflux disease (GERD) need to not only avoid acidic foods but also avoid foods that loosen the lower esophageal sphincter and cause more digestive backflow, such as large quantities of high-fat meals.

The Bottom Line: The alkaline diet is suggested for acid reflux because the saturated fat in foods such as meats and cheeses causes digestive delay. The alkaline diet also avoids foods that can aggravate acid reflux, such as dairy, garlic, and tomatoes. Note that foods such as lemons, limes, and oranges are considered alkaline but can actually be detrimental to someone with GERD because the acid content does not get neutralized until it reaches the stomach.

Weight Loss

The alkaline diet was made famous by its celebrity followers, including Victoria Beckham, Kelly Ripa, and Jennifer Aniston. Followers of the alkaline diet claim that eating acidic foods causes the body to hold on to excess fat.

What We Know: Weight gain and obesity can be a result of hormonal imbalance, insulin resistance, excess calorie intake, and many more factors. Following a Western diet that is abundant in processed foods, sugar, and animal-based protein can have negative effects on your hormones and lead to insulin resistance and eating too many non-nutritive calories.

The Bottom Line: Following a diet that is high in fruits and vegetables has been shown to lead to weight loss due to its nutritional content and not necessarily due to its alkalinity. The high amount of fiber in plant-based diets also leads to a greater feeling of satiety and positive changes in the gut microbiome.

Blood Pressure

According to the World Health Organization, about 1.13 billion people around the world have high blood pressure. The proponents of the alkaline diet believe that eating more plant-based foods helps lower blood pressure.

What We Know: Studies have shown that a diet high in fruits, vegetables, and legumes can reduce blood pressure but not due to its alkaline properties. The high potassium content in these foods helps maintain the body's sodium balance and helps temporarily widen the blood vessels (vasodilation), which aids in blood pressure control. The Dietary Approaches to Stop Hypertension (DASH) diet is considered an effective way to lower blood pressure.

The Bottom Line: Both the DASH diet and the alkaline diet focus on eating more foods that are rich in antioxidants, potassium, and fiber, which has been shown to benefit overall cardiovascular function.

Depression and Mood

Globally, about 300 million people suffer from depression. But we can assume that the number is actually much higher. The proponents of the alkaline diet believe that food directly affects our mood.

What We Know: Our microbiome (all the microbes that live on and inside the human body) is closely connected to our central nervous system; this is known as the gut-brain axis. An imbalance of gut microbiota can significantly affect brain development and functioning via the gut-brain axis—which includes the neural, endocrine, and immune pathways.

The Bottom Line: The alkaline diet includes lots of prebiotic foods that serve as fertilizer for good gut bacteria. Without whole grains such as oats, fruits, and vegetables, probiotics (your good gut bacteria) can't flourish.

Cardiovascular Disease

Cardiovascular disease includes high blood pressure, atherosclerosis, ischemic heart disease, peripheral vascular disease, and heart failure. It is associated with fatty plaque buildup in the arteries. The proponents of the alkaline diet believe that by eliminating or reducing intake of animal protein and eating more fresh produce, you can lower heart disease risk factors.

What We Know: Research suggests that following a Mediterranean diet that is high in fruits, vegetables, whole grains, fish, and extra-virgin olive oil and low in processed foods has been effective in preventing cardiovascular disease. Like the Mediterranean diet, the alkaline diet focuses on limiting processed foods and consuming mostly plant-based, dairy-free foods.

The Bottom Line: Conclusive research states that following a diet that is high in vegetables, fruit, whole grains, and legumes and limiting added sugars, processed foods, red meat, and processed meat decreases the risk of developing a variety of health conditions. The nutritional balance in food, rather than its alkalinity or acidity, has an effect on preventing and treating many diseases.

What to Eat and Avoid

The alkaline diet proposes that when food is eaten and converted into energy, one of the byproducts is ash residue, which is either acidic or alkaline. Foods that are alkaline retain a pH of 8 to 14 in the body, and foods that are acidic retain a pH of 0 to 6. Although science does not back up the acid-ash hypothesis, a whole-food, plant-based, dairy-free diet is widely recognized to aid overall health and help prevent disease.

What to Eat

In this book, alkaline foods are plant-based foods that contain a wide variety of essential vitamins, minerals, amino acids, and antioxidants. Here are the specific foods that I recommend.

Dark, leafy greens: Greens like kale, spinach, chard, and arugula are high in vitamins A, C, and K as well as folate, fiber, magnesium, calcium, iron, and potassium.

Extra-virgin olive oil and avocado oil: High in monounsaturated and polyunsaturated fats, these healthy oils benefit the brain, nerves, skin, nails, and hormonal regulation.

Fruits: Studies show that eating fruit is related to a lower risk of diabetes. Blueberries, cherries, apples, and raspberries are especially rich in fiber and antioxidants.

Legumes: Legumes are high in protein, iron, B vitamins, folic acid, fiber, and unsaturated fatty acids. Choose from a wide variety, including lentils, chickpeas, lima beans, black-eyed peas, and mung beans.

Non-starchy vegetables: Known to lower blood pressure and cancer risk, these vegetables can also provide a favorable ratio of sodium to potassium, which may reduce urinary calcium loss and benefit bone health. Examples are radishes, mushrooms, artichokes, asparagus, broccoli, cauliflower, cucumber, carrots, jicama, peppers, and leafy greens.

Nuts: Almonds, cashews, macadamia nuts, Brazil nuts, and other nuts are high in healthy unsaturated, monounsaturated, and polyunsaturated fatty acids.

Seeds: Seeds are high in antioxidants, healthy fat, fiber, and omega 3 fatty acids. Chia, hemp, and flax seeds are examples.

Soybeans: Soybeans, such as edamame and tofu, contain essential amino acids and are high in protein, making them a great substitute for animal proteins.

Whole grains: Whole grains, like quinoa, buckwheat, and brown rice, contain iron, magnesium, and phosphorus. They also provide complex carbohydrates and are high in fiber, which aids in blood sugar control.

What to Avoid

Added sugars: Eating too much added sugar has been linked to weight gain, insulin resistance, cardiovascular problems, inflammation, blood platelet disruption, and oxidative stress. Examples of sugar include brown sugar, refined white sugar, rice syrup, dextrose, honey, malt sugar, and molasses.

Alcohol: Alcohol contains empty calories that do not contribute to overall health and contribute to weight gain. Excessive alcohol intake is associated with heart disease, liver damage, and high blood pressure, as well as dehydration and malnutrition.

Dairy: Dairy products, including milk, butter, kefir, yogurt, and ice cream, are known to cause allergies or sensitivities, and evidence supports a potential link to higher levels of inflammation.

Fish and seafood: Of all the animal-based protein sources, fish provides the most health benefits. Fish is high in omega 3 fatty acids, which are powerful sources of antioxidants that have been shown to improve cardiovascular health. However, fish is acidic, so when following an alkaline diet, you can include fish in moderation, following the 80/20 approach (see page 12).

Highly processed grains: Highly processed grains can take the form of cookies, chips, muffins, crackers, tortillas, cakes, crackers, and pastries. They contain toxic additives such as sugars, chemicals, and stabilizers.

Poultry: Poultry such as chicken, turkey, and duck are all considered acidic. Although chicken and turkey are commonly considered lean meats, they are still associated with an increased risk of cardiovascular disease.

Processed meats: These are meats like sausage, bacon, ham, and hot dogs that are preserved by smoking, curing, salting, or adding chemical preservatives. Eating a lot of these meats has been linked to heart disease, high blood pressure, and cancer.

Protein supplements: Protein powders and protein bars often contain added sugars, gums, and additives. The protein sources are often highly processed. Choose protein from whole foods instead.

Red meat: Meats such as beef, pork, veal, and lamb are high in saturated fat, which correlates with cardiovascular disease risks. The evidence linking red meat consumption with cancer is generally consistent.

THE 80/20 APPROACH

About 95 percent of diets fail, and most people regain most or all of the weight lost because our relationship with food cannot be changed overnight. A restrictive diet almost always leads to feeling deprived, resulting in binge eating of the very foods we want to avoid and a preoccupation with food.

What I like about the alkaline diet is that it follows the 80/20 rule. With the 80/20 approach, you can eat alkaline foods 80 percent of the time. The remaining 20 percent makes room for acidic foods to keep your diet realistic and sustainable. Nutritious acidic foods that you can enjoy occasionally include popcorn, wild-caught fish, grass-fed steak, peanut butter, and even a glass of wine.

Setting Up Your Kitchen

Perhaps you're wondering if you should start eating more alkaline foods after you finish all the processed foods in your pantry. There is no need to do more harm to your body before trying to heal it! The first step in following the alkaline diet is setting yourself up for success. Let's get your kitchen organized so that it's stocked with plenty of alkaline foods you can enjoy any time.

Refrigerator Essentials

- Berries
- Fresh herbs: parsley, mint, cilantro
- Ginger
- Kale
- Lemon
- Medjool dates
- Miso
- Mushrooms
- Onions
- Zucchini

Pantry Essentials

- Agave syrup
- Apple cider vinegar
- Coconut milk: full-fat, canned
- Grains: quinoa, wild rice, oats
- Lentils
- Nuts
- Oils: olive, coconut, and avocado*
- Seeds: sesame, flax, chia, pumpkin, sunflower
- Spices: cumin, cinnamon, turmeric
- Tahini

*I recommend extra-virgin olive oil for low-heat cooking and for dressings, due to its low smoke point. For high-heat cooking such as baking, roasting, or frying, I suggest using coconut oil or avocado oil, which have a high smoke point.

Basic Kitchen Equipment

The following basic, affordable kitchen equipment will help you prepare recipes easily.

Blender: You will use your blender a lot for the recipes in chapters 3 and 4. You can use a small single-serve blender or a high-speed countertop blender. A single-serve blender is usually less money than a countertop blender, but if you use it to make soups, you may need to blend the soups in batches.

Can opener: This is a must-have tool because you will be cooking with canned products such as beans and coconut milk. You can use dried beans, of course, but canned beans can be more convenient when you're in a hurry.

Measuring spoons and cups: Since you will be trying new recipes in this book, measuring cups and spoons are a must. Following the recipes correctly will ensure that your food is delicious!

Miniature food processor: This is one of my favorite kitchen tools. I use it to chop vegetables, make sauces, and much more. It is easy to wash and store.

Pots and pans: The recipes in this book call for a medium saucepan (4-quart), a large Dutch oven or stockpot (6- to 8-quart), and a nonstick or cast-iron skillet (10- to 12-inch).

Rimmed baking sheets (2): Baking sheets let you not only roast vegetables beautifully but also help when it comes to making one-pot (or -pan) meals. If you already have the oven turned on to make dinner, that's a great opportunity to prep your next meal by roasting a second pan of vegetables.

About the Recipes

Making positive changes doesn't have to be complicated. In working with my nutrition clients—and cooking for my family of four—I've learned that the simpler the recipe, the better. But simple does not have to mean flavorless or boring, especially if you are working with high-quality, in-season ingredients.

All the recipes in this book have five ingredients or less, not including water, oil, salt, and pepper, and all the ingredients are easy to find. Many of these recipes fall into one of two categories of ease, indicated by the following icons:

 One-pot. Recipes that require only one cooking vessel to make.

 30-minute. Recipes that take less than 30 minutes to prepare and cook (more than three-quarters of the recipes in this book!).

All the recipes in this book are 100 percent alkaline meals, so they can be a reliable alkaline food resource. For the 20 percent acidic foods, focus on complementing your alkaline foods. For example, since the majority of alkaline foods are fruits and vegetables, try to add acidic foods that supply essential nutrients that could be lacking in plant-based diets, such as B vitamins, iron, calcium, and vitamin D. When you are dining out or celebrating a special occasion, your 20 percent can be a slice of cake or even a glass of wine.

Finally, the most important part of this journey is to focus on what you should be eating more of, rather than foods you should avoid. When you shift your focus to what you're adding, instead of what you're taking away, you're more likely to stick to your good health journey.

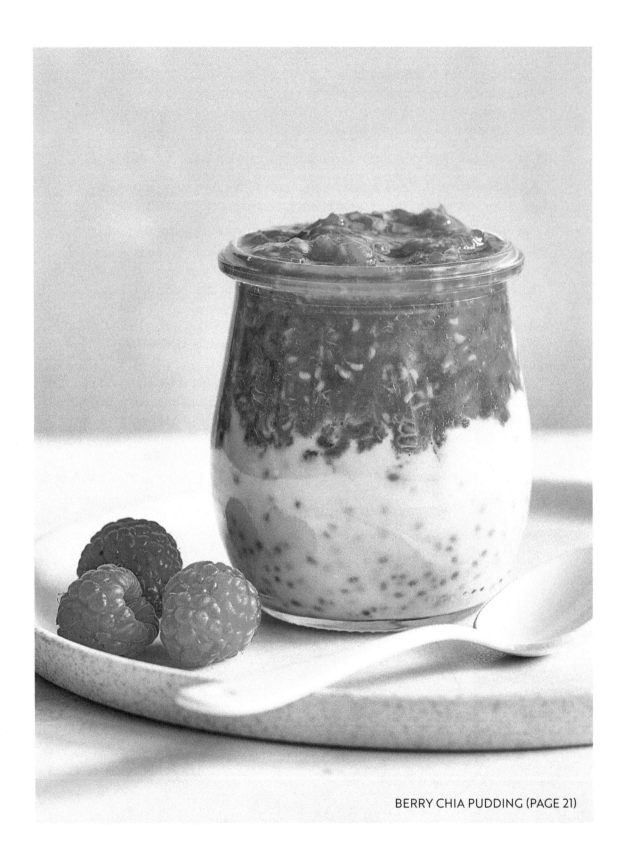

BERRY CHIA PUDDING (PAGE 21)

Breakfasts

• • • • •

Coconut Yogurt Parfait

SERVES 2 • **PREP TIME:** 5 MINUTES

As a busy working mom of two kids, I am a big fan of easy breakfasts that require no cooking and fewer dirty dishes. This yogurt parfait comes together in less than 5 minutes. The flavor of coconut yogurt and banana work well with the chia seeds, which are packed with fiber to make this breakfast satisfying. Coconut yogurt is high in medium chain triglycerides (MCT), a kind of fatty acid that's quick and easy for the body to turn into energy and that may be helpful for weight loss.

1½ cups plain coconut yogurt

1 medium banana, peeled and cut into ½-inch coins

1 tablespoon chia seeds

2 tablespoons cashew butter

Put the coconut yogurt in a serving bowl, and top with the banana, chia seeds, and cashew butter. Serve immediately.

VARIATION TIP: Try this recipe with other alkaline fruits or nuts, such as peaches, macadamia nuts, and hemp seeds.

PER SERVING: Calories: 293; Fat: 17g; Protein: 3g; Carbohydrates: 38g; Fiber: 8.5g; Sodium: 9mg; Iron: 2mg

Breakfast Banana Split

SERVES 2 • **PREP TIME:** 5 MINUTES

This is a more nutritionally balanced version of ants on a log (typically peanut butter, celery, and raisins). Bananas are high in vitamin B_6, which is more often found in protein-rich foods like turkey and beans. Vitamin B_6 also plays an important role in mood regulation, nutrient metabolism, and even creating neurotransmitters. If you are worried about the sugar content of the banana, reduce the portion size or pair it with high-fat or high-protein ingredients to balance out the sugar, as I did with this recipe.

2 bananas, peeled

2 tablespoons almond butter

2 tablespoons hemp hearts

2 tablespoons unsweetened coconut flakes

1. Cut the bananas in half lengthwise.
2. Spread ½ tablespoon of almond butter on each half of each banana and sprinkle with the hemp hearts and coconut flakes.

VARIATION TIP: You can also use cashew butter (my favorite!) or different seeds, such as chia seeds and flax seeds, to add variety.

PER SERVING: Calories: 282; Fat: 15g; Protein: 8g; Carbohydrates: 32g; Fiber: 6g; Sodium: 37mg; Iron: 2.5mg

Coconut-Mango Chia Pudding

SERVES 2 • **PREP TIME:** 5 MINUTES, PLUS 15 MINUTES TO THICKEN

I started making this coconut chia pudding for my daughter when she was five months old, and today it is a family favorite. The chia seeds add extra fiber and omega 3s. Fiber is crucial for gut health and blood sugar regulation, and omega 3 fatty acids have excellent anti-inflammatory properties. Make extra batches and keep them in your refrigerator for up to three or four days.

3 tablespoons chia seeds

1 cup canned full-fat coconut milk

1 cup minced fresh or frozen mango

1. In a pint-size jar, mix together the chia seeds, coconut milk, and mango. Seal with an airtight lid.
2. Chill the jar in the refrigerator for about 15 minutes before serving.

MAKE AHEAD TIP: You can keep the pudding in your refrigerator for up to 7 days if you make it without the fruit. Then just add fresh fruit when you are ready to serve.

VARIATION TIP: Try this recipe with other alkaline fruits, such as pineapple—one of my favorites!

PER SERVING: Calories: 348; Fat: 29g; Protein: 5g; Carbohydrates: 22g; Fiber: 8g; Sodium: 18mg; Iron: 5mg

Berry Chia Pudding

SERVES 2 • **PREP TIME:** 5 MINUTES, PLUS 15 MINUTES TO THICKEN

Chia seeds are packed with so many nutrients! Two tablespoons of chia seeds have as much fiber as 10 cups of raw spinach. They're also high in protein, omega 3 fatty acids, magnesium, calcium, and antioxidants, which help fight free radicals that contribute to cancers and aging.

3 tablespoons
chia seeds

1 cup unsweetened
almond milk

1 tablespoon
agave syrup

1 cup raspberries,
mashed

1. In a pint-size jar, mix the chia seeds, almond milk, and agave syrup well. Seal with an airtight lid.
2. Refrigerate the pudding for at least 15 minutes or leave it overnight to thicken.
3. Add the mashed raspberries and serve cold.

VARIATION TIP: Add ground chia seeds instead if you don't like the texture of whole chia seeds.

PER SERVING: Calories: 158; Fat: 6.5g; Protein: 4g; Carbohydrates: 23g; Fiber: 9.5g; Sodium: 96mg; Iron: 3mg

Apple-Cashew Cold Porridge

SERVES 4 • **PREP TIME:** 10 MINUTES

This cold porridge requires just your blender, making it perfect for a summer morning. Inspired by Cafe Gratitude in Venice, California (one of my favorite restaurants), this recipe is an alkaline version of their Apple-Pecan Porridge. This well-balanced breakfast has healthy fats from coconut milk, protein from cashews, and carbohydrates from an apple. It's sure to keep you energized and full until lunchtime.

1 large apple, cored and coarsely chopped

½ cup frozen pineapple chunks

2½ cups canned full-fat coconut milk

⅓ cup raw cashews

½ teaspoon ground cinnamon, plus more as needed

⅛ teaspoon kosher salt

1. Put the apple, pineapple, coconut milk, cashews, and cinnamon in a high-speed blender.
2. Pulse for about 10 seconds until the mixture resembles a chunky porridge.
3. Pour the porridge into 2 bowls and sprinkle with the salt and additional cinnamon as desired.

INGREDIENT TIP: I left out vanilla extract to make this recipe 100 percent alkaline, but you can add ¼ teaspoon vanilla seeds if you'd like.

PER SERVING: Calories: 373; Fat: 34g; Protein: 5g; Carbohydrates: 17g; Fiber: 3.5g; Sodium: 93mg; Iron: 5.5mg

Coconut-Cashew Cold Porridge

SERVES 4 • **PREP TIME:** 5 MINUTES

Did I mention how easy it is to prepare this crunchy and refreshing breakfast porridge? It's similar to a smoothie, but rather than blending it until smooth, you blend just enough to get the ingredients chunky and thick, so there's more texture. Top with strawberries if they're in season.

1 large apple, cored and coarsely chopped

2½ cups full-fat coconut milk

⅓ cup raw cashews

½ teaspoon ground cinnamon

⅛ **teaspoon kosher salt**

Put the apple, coconut milk, cashews, cinnamon, and salt in a blender. Blend until the mixture is chunky, resembling the consistency of oatmeal. Serve cold.

VARIATION TIP: Think of the apple, coconut milk, and nuts as your base for this porridge, and add any other ingredients you like to create something new.

PER SERVING: Calories: 361; Fat: 34g; Protein: 4g; Carbohydrates: 14g; Fiber: 3.5g; Sodium: 56mg; Iron: 5.5mg

Apple-Cinnamon Oatmeal

SERVES 2 • **PREP TIME:** 5 MINUTES • **COOK TIME:** 5 MINUTES

One of the few grains that are alkaline diet friendly, oats are easy to cook and nutritionally balanced with carbohydrates, fat, fiber, and protein. They're also a great prebiotic, working as a fertilizer for the good bacteria in your gut. In fact, they have been shown to be beneficial for blood sugar control and lowering cholesterol. This recipe works well with fruit but can also become savory with your favorite herbs and spices.

⅔ cup old-fashioned rolled oats or quick-cooking oatmeal

1½ cups unsweetened almond milk

1 small apple, cored and chopped into ½-inch cubes

⅓ teaspoon ground cinnamon

1. In a small pot, bring the oats and almond milk to a simmer.
2. Add the apple and cook, stirring constantly, for 3 to 5 minutes or until the oatmeal looks creamy.
3. Transfer the oatmeal to 2 bowls and add the cinnamon.

MAKE AHEAD TIP: This recipe can be prepared ahead and will keep in the refrigerator for about 2 or 3 days.

INGREDIENT TIP: Instant oatmeal cooks much faster than old-fashioned rolled oats. If you are using the instant oatmeal, you can microwave it instead of cooking it over the stove.

PER SERVING: Calories: 170; Fat: 4.5g; Protein: 5g; Carbohydrates: 30g; Fiber: 4.5g; Sodium: 140mg; Iron: 2mg

Quinoa-Apricot Porridge

SERVES 2 • **PREP TIME:** 5 MINUTES • **COOK TIME:** 5 MINUTES

Apricots are rich in vitamin A and beta carotene, which are antioxidants that protect your cells from damage. I love making this porridge in the summer when apricots are super juicy and sweet. When cooked, summer apricots become delightfully jam-like and pair well with the nutty quinoa. You can also make this with oatmeal, but the quinoa adds a nice texture. In the summer, this can be made in advance and served cold as a breakfast or a snack.

½ cup cooked quinoa

1¼ cups unsweetened almond milk

2 fresh apricots, pitted and finely chopped

¼ teaspoon ground cinnamon

2 tablespoons chopped raw almonds

1. In a small saucepan, combine the quinoa, almond milk, and apricots. Bring to a simmer over medium heat. Cook, stirring frequently, for 3 to 5 minutes, or until the mixture comes to a boil.
2. Divide the mixture into 2 serving bowls and sprinkle with the cinnamon and chopped almonds. Serve immediately.

   INGREDIENT TIP: To cook quinoa, rinse it thoroughly, then combine 1 part uncooked quinoa and 2 parts water, and simmer for 10 minutes. Cooked quinoa will keep in the refrigerator for several days.

   VARIATION TIP: Try adding 1 tablespoon almond butter, 1 tablespoon chia seeds, or your favorite oatmeal topping.

PER SERVING: Calories: 136; Fat: 6g; Protein: 5g; Carbohydrates: 16g; Fiber: 3g; Sodium: 120mg; Iron: 1.5mg

Everyday Granola

MAKES 4 CUPS • PREP TIME: 5 MINUTES • COOK TIME: 20 MINUTES

Unlike store-bought granolas, which are usually high in sugar and full of additives, this homemade granola is packed with nutrients such as vitamin E and selenium. Vitamin E protects your cells against the negative effects of free radicals, and selenium is important for your immune system. Most importantly, it is crunchy, nutty, and so easy to make. Prepare a large batch to have enough for a few weeks and to give as gifts to friends and family.

1 cup old-fashioned rolled oats

1 cup sunflower seeds

2 cups raw almonds

2 tablespoons coconut oil, melted

¼ cup agave syrup

½ teaspoon kosher salt

1. Preheat the oven to 350°F. Line a baking sheet with parchment paper.
2. In a large mixing bowl, combine the oats, sunflower seeds, almonds, coconut oil, and agave syrup. Mix well.
3. Transfer the mixture to the prepared baking sheet and bake for 20 minutes, turning the baking sheet halfway through.
4. Let granola cool completely, then sprinkle with the salt.

MAKE AHEAD TIP: This recipe can be made in a large batch and stored in an airtight container for up to 2 weeks.

VARIATION TIP: You can add ⅓ cup sesame seeds to make this extra nutty.

PER SERVING (⅓ CUP): Calories: 260; Fat: 19g; Protein: 8g; Carbohydrates: 17g; Fiber: 4.5g; Sodium: 47mg; Iron: 2mg

Grain-Free Granola

MAKES 3 CUPS • **PREP TIME:** 5 MINUTES • **COOK TIME:** 15 MINUTES

This versatile grain-free granola is crunchy, nutty, and perfect on your salad, oatmeal, fresh fruits, and even on coconut yogurt. Plant-based fats from nuts and seeds are excellent sources of omega 3 fatty acids, which help reduce inflammation in your body. Additionally, nuts are high in protein and fiber, which are crucial for energy and gut health. You can also add old-fashioned rolled oats and freeze-dried strawberries to jazz up this dish.

1 cup raw cashews, coarsely chopped

1 cup raw sliced almonds

½ cup pumpkin seeds

½ cup sunflower seeds

3 tablespoons agave syrup

¼ cup extra-virgin olive oil

1 teaspoon kosher salt

1. Preheat the oven to 350°F. Line a large baking sheet with parchment paper.
2. In a large mixing bowl, combine the cashews, almonds, pumpkin seeds, sunflower seeds, agave syrup, and olive oil.
3. Spread the mixture evenly on the prepared baking sheet and bake for 15 minutes, stirring halfway through.
4. Let granola cool completely, then sprinkle with the salt.

   VARIATION TIP: Use coconut oil instead of olive oil for a different flavor.

PER SERVING (⅓ CUP): Calories: 302; Fat: 25g; Protein: 9g; Carbohydrates: 13g; Fiber: 3.5g; Sodium: 127mg; Iron: 3mg

Baked Oatmeal Bars

MAKES 8 BARS • **PREP TIME:** 10 MINUTES • **COOK TIME:** 30 MINUTES

My family loves these bars as a quick breakfast or snack. You can add your favorite nuts or even dried fruits to make them even more delicious. Turn this into a quick dessert by serving it with a scoop of vegan ice cream and some chopped nuts.

Extra-virgin olive oil

2 tablespoons flaxseed meal

5 tablespoons water

½ cup plain pumpkin puree

1 teaspoon ground cinnamon

2½ cups old-fashioned rolled oats

2 cups full-fat coconut milk

1. Preheat the oven to 350°F. Grease a 2-quart baking dish with olive oil.
2. In a large mixing bowl, combine the flaxseed meal and water. Set it aside for 2 or 3 minutes to thicken. Add the pumpkin puree, cinnamon, oats, and coconut milk. Mix well to combine.
3. Transfer the mixture to the prepared baking dish and spread evenly. Bake for 30 minutes or until the top is golden brown.
4. Let cool completely before cutting into 8 bars.

MAKE AHEAD TIP: These bars keep in the refrigerator for up to 3 days and up to 1 month in the freezer.

PER SERVING (1 BAR): Calories: 250; Fat: 18g; Protein: 5g; Carbohydrates: 20g; Fiber: 4g; Sodium: 8mg; Iron: 3mg

Flaxseed-Banana Muffins

MAKES 12 MUFFINS • **PREP TIME:** 10 MINUTES • **COOK TIME:** 20 MINUTES

When you're following a specific diet for your health, you want to set yourself up for success by having plenty of ready-to-eat meals prepared. These muffins are great when you're craving a starchy breakfast or snack. I love to add fresh blueberries to the batter to make blueberry muffins. These muffins pair well with simple mashed raspberries as jam.

1 tablespoon coconut oil

2 tablespoons flaxseed meal

6 tablespoons water

2 cups old-fashioned rolled oats

3 ripe bananas, peeled and mashed

2 tablespoons agave syrup

1 teaspoon baking soda

1. Preheat the oven to 350°F. Grease a 12-cup muffin tin with the coconut oil.
2. In a large mixing bowl, combine the flaxseed meal and water. Let it thicken for 2 to 3 minutes.
3. Add the oats, bananas, agave syrup, and baking soda to the flaxseed mixture. Mix well.
4. Pour the batter into the muffin tin and bake for 20 minutes, or until a toothpick inserted in to the center of a muffin comes out clean.

MAKE AHEAD TIP: Make the muffins ahead, and store half of them in the freezer and the other half in the refrigerator in airtight containers. They can be warmed up quickly in the microwave for 15 to 30 seconds.

INGREDIENT TIP: Flaxseed meal is a great substitute for eggs when baking things like muffins.

PER SERVING (1 MUFFIN): Calories: 102; Fat: 2.5g; Protein: 2g; Carbohydrates: 19g; Fiber: 2.5g; Sodium: 105mg; Iron: 1mg

Vegan Banana Pancakes

MAKES 6 MINI PANCAKES • **PREP TIME:** 5 MINUTES • **COOK TIME:** 10 MINUTES

My family's go-to breakfast, these delicious pancakes require just four ingredients and are super simple to make. You can use canned coconut milk instead of almond milk to make this heartier. I like to add a hint of cinnamon to the batter for warmth and sweetness. If I am expecting a particularly chaotic day, I prepare the batter the night before and make the pancakes in the morning.

1 ripe banana, peeled

1 cup old-fashioned rolled oats or instant oatmeal

½ cup unsweetened almond milk

¼ teaspoon ground cinnamon

1. In a large mixing bowl, mash the banana with a fork until it's slightly lumpy but mostly creamy. Add the oats, almond milk, and cinnamon.
2. Heat a large nonstick skillet over medium heat.
3. Add 1½ tablespoons of the batter to the skillet for each pancake.
4. Cook the pancakes for about 2 to 4 minutes, then flip and cook for 2 minutes on the other side. Serve immediately.

MAKE AHEAD TIP: The batter can be prepared up to 24 hours in advance. Store it in an airtight container in the refrigerator.

VARIATION TIP: Add chopped almonds to the batter, or serve the pancakes with almond or cashew butter alongside fresh raspberries.

PER SERVING (3 PANCAKES): Calories: 212; Fat: 4g; Protein: 6g; Carbohydrates: 41g; Fiber: 5.5g; Sodium: 47mg; Iron: 2mg

Leek and Kale Scramble

SERVES 2 • **PREP TIME:** 5 MINUTES • **COOK TIME:** 10 MINUTES

Leeks contain high amounts of a type of antioxidant called flavonoids. Flavonoids protect your body by fighting against free radicals that can cause oxidative damage. Leeks have a milder flavor than onions and are delicious when caramelized. If you enjoy them, try the Steamed Leeks with Mustard Vinaigrette (page 62).

2 tablespoons extra-virgin olive oil

1 cup thinly sliced leeks

3 cups baby kale

1½ cups grated zucchini

1 tablespoon caraway seeds

⅓ teaspoon ground ginger

⅓ teaspoon kosher salt

⅓ teaspoon freshly ground black pepper

1. In a large skillet, heat the olive oil over medium-high heat.
2. Add the leeks and sauté for about 3 minutes, until they're lightly browned.
3. Add the kale, zucchini, caraway seeds, ginger, salt, and pepper. Cook for about 5 minutes, or until the vegetables are cooked through. Serve warm.

VARIATION TIP: This makes a great base for a shakshuka. Simply add eggs at the end of step 3, cover, and let sit until the egg whites are cooked. Since eggs are acidic, you can add ⅓ cup cooked lentils to keep the recipe alkaline.

PER SERVING: Calories: 106; Fat: 5.5g; Protein: 4g; Carbohydrates: 12g; Fiber: 4.5g; Sodium: 182mg; Iron: 2.5mg

Sweet Potato Hash

SERVES 2 • **PREP TIME:** 5 MINUTES • **COOK TIME:** 10 MINUTES

Purple sweet potatoes are high in anthocyanin, a powerful antioxidant that fights free radicals and offers anti-inflammatory and antiviral benefits. Orange sweet potatoes are rich in beta carotene, another antioxidant. Sweet potatoes are also high in fiber and vitamin C, making this breakfast not only delicious but also nutrient packed. If you are feeling hungrier than usual, add ¼ cup cooked edamame for more protein and fiber.

2 tablespoons extra-virgin olive oil

2 large purple or orange sweet potatoes, peeled and spiralized

⅛ teaspoon kosher salt

⅛ teaspoon freshly ground black pepper

¼ cup chopped fresh parsley

1. In a large skillet, heat the olive oil over medium-high heat. When the oil is hot, add the sweet potatoes.
2. Add the salt and pepper. Sauté for 5 to 7 minutes or until the sweet potatoes are tender and lightly browned.
3. Serve warm, topped with the chopped parsley.

INGREDIENT TIP: If you don't have a spiralizer, you can simply cut your sweet potatoes into ½-inch cubes.

PER SERVING: Calories: 248; Fat: 13g; Protein: 2g; Carbohydrates: 30g; Fiber: 4.5g; Sodium: 155mg; Iron: 1.5mg

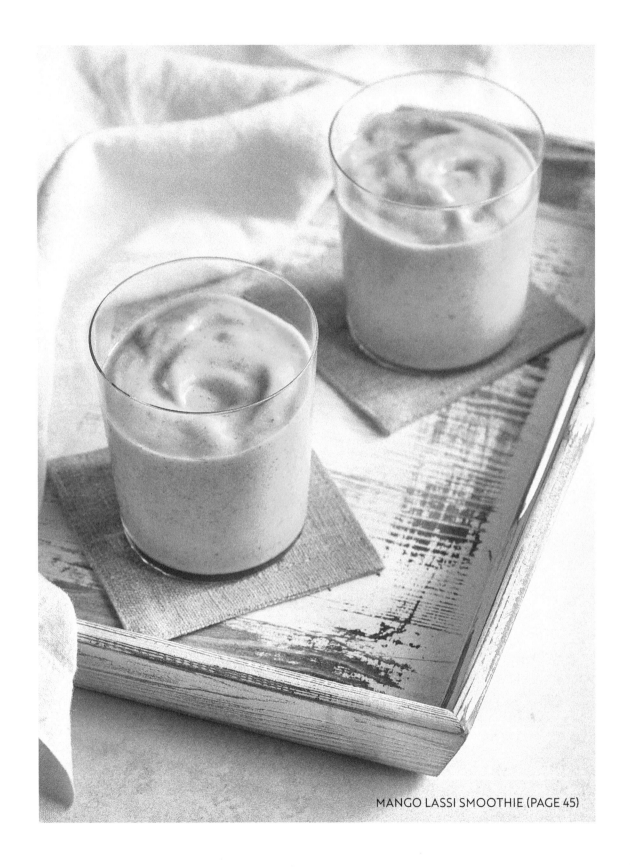

MANGO LASSI SMOOTHIE (PAGE 45)

Juices and Smoothies

• • • • •

Everyday Green Juice

SERVES 2 • **PREP TIME:** 5 MINUTES

I love making green juice with my son on weekends. I get to hand over the vegetables to him, and he gets to feed the juicer. Because I share my green juice with my toddler, I try not to add too many fruits and stick to lemon and ginger for flavor. Fruit juices are low in fiber and high in sugar, so they can cause a significant spike in blood sugar levels, leading to inflammation in your body. Fruits with less sugar, like lemon and lime, can add so much flavor without having a big impact on your blood sugar.

1 bunch celery

4 cups kale

1 large seedless cucumber

1 lemon

1 thumb-size piece fresh ginger

1. Clean and coarsely chop the celery, kale, cucumber, lemon, and ginger. (The lemon and ginger can be juiced with skin on or off.)
2. Juice the celery, kale, cucumber, lemon, and ginger.
3. If you don't have a juicer, put all the ingredients in a blender and blend until everything is liquefied. Strain the juice through a fine-mesh colander or a piece of cheesecloth.

INGREDIENT TIP: The vitamins in fresh juices like this one can oxidize easily, so they should be consumed immediately or stored in an airtight container in the refrigerator for up to 24 hours.

PER SERVING: Calories: 71; Fat: 0.5g; Protein: 4g; Carbohydrates: 14g; Fiber: 7g; Sodium: 172mg; Iron: 1.5mg

Glow Cooler

This refreshing cooler is the perfect midday drink to give you the energy you need to get on with the rest of your day. Aloe has antioxidant properties, alleviates heartburn, aids in digestion, and is a great source of vitamin C and magnesium. Due to its rich antioxidant content, aloe can help prevent many chronic diseases brought about by oxidative stress.

2 cups water

1 cup ice cubes

2 tablespoons aloe vera juice or 2 tablespoons fresh aloe vera

1 cup kale

½ cup fresh or frozen pineapple chunks

1 pitted Medjool date

1. Put the water, ice, aloe vera, kale, pineapple, and date in a blender. Blend until the mixture is smooth and creamy.
2. Serve immediately or store in an airtight container in the refrigerator for up to 24 hours.

PER SERVING: Calories: 47; Fat: 0g; Protein: 1g; Carbohydrates: 12g; Fiber: 1.5g; Sodium: 4mg; Iron: 0.5mg

Watermelon Cooler

SERVES 2 • **PREP TIME:** 5 MINUTES

Every time my son eats his favorite fruits, he asks if we can make juice out of them. Sometimes we juice them to see what they look and taste like, but most of the time I like to blend them for him so that he can enjoy his favorite fruits without leaving all the fiber behind. Try this watermelon cooler on a hot summer day and make ice pops with any leftovers.

4 cups seedless watermelon cubes

10 fresh mint leaves

1 tablespoon agave syrup

1 cup ice cubes

Put the watermelon, mint, agave syrup, and ice in a blender. Blend until the watermelon has liquefied. Serve immediately.

MAKE AHEAD TIP: If you are making this recipe ahead, you can make it without ice and add the ice when you're ready to drink it.

PER SERVING: Calories: 121; Fat: 0.5g; Protein: 2g; Carbohydrates: 31g; Fiber: 1g; Sodium: 3mg; Iron: 1.5mg

Black Sesame Milk

I grew up drinking black sesame milk. My mom used to say that black sesame makes your gray hair go away. That certainly has not happened yet, but I still enjoy making this super creamy sesame milk. Just one pitted date adds a hint of sweetness to this milk. Serve cold or warm, depending on the weather.

1 cup black sesame seeds, soaked overnight and drained

4 cups water

1 pitted Medjool date

⅛ **teaspoon kosher salt**

1. Put the soaked and drained black sesame seeds, water, date, and salt in a blender. Blend on high speed for about 60 seconds.
2. Strain the mixture through a fine-mesh sieve or a nut milk bag into a large bowl, discarding the solids.
3. Transfer the liquid to an airtight container and refrigerate until you're ready to serve.

MAKE AHEAD TIP: This recipe can be prepared in a large batch and stored in an airtight container for 3 to 4 days in the refrigerator.

PER SERVING: Calories: 218; Fat: 18g; Protein: 8g; Carbohydrates: 22g; Fiber: 4g; Sodium: 39mg; Iron: 4mg

Creamy Cashew Milk

This cashew milk is a staple in my household. I make a big batch every week to add to smoothies, drink cold on its own, or warm up with one or two cardamom pods to make spiced lattes. Homemade plant-based milk is free of artificial flavors and additives such as thickeners that have been shown to irritate your gut. But most importantly, homemade is way more delicious.

1 cup raw
unsalted cashews

4 cups water

½ teaspoon ground
cinnamon

⅛ **teaspoon kosher salt**

1. Soak the cashews in a bowl of warm water for 30 minutes, then drain.
2. Put the drained cashews, water, cinnamon, and salt in a blender. Blend for about 60 seconds on high speed, or until the mixture is smooth.
3. Transfer the mixture to an airtight container and store in the refrigerator for up to 4 days.

INGREDIENT TIP: You can skip the soaking if you are short on time. Just blend everything for about 15 seconds longer to achieve a creamy consistency.

PER SERVING: Calories: 161; Fat: 12g; Protein: 5g; Carbohydrates: 8g; Fiber: 1g; Sodium: 40mg; Iron: 2mg

Bright-Eyed Blueberry Smoothie

SERVES 2 • PREP TIME: 5 MINUTES

According to my husband, this smoothie tastes more like Oreo cookies than a blueberry smoothie. It's nutty, creamy, and refreshing—a perfect way to start your morning. My new clients often tell me that smoothies make them hungrier. That's likely true if the smoothie is low in protein and fiber. The chia seeds, nut butter, and higher-fiber fruit in this recipe will keep you full and give you lasting energy to start your day off right.

1 cup water

1 cup ice cubes

1 cup unsweetened almond milk

1 cup frozen blueberries

2 cups baby spinach

2 tablespoons chia seeds

2 tablespoons almond butter

1. Put the water, ice, almond milk, blueberries, spinach, chia seeds, and almond butter in a blender. Blend until the mixture is creamy and smooth.
2. Divide the smoothie between 2 serving glasses and serve immediately.

MAKE AHEAD TIP: This smoothie can be made in advance and kept in the freezer for up to 1 week or in the refrigerator for up to 24 hours.

HEALTH TIP: Blueberries contain anthocyanins, a powerful antioxidant that may protect your retinas from oxidative stress.

PER SERVING: Calories: 214; Fat: 13g; Protein: 7g; Carbohydrates: 18g; Fiber: 8.5g; Sodium: 176mg; Iron: 3.5mg

Mango, Kale, and Ginger Smoothie

SERVES 2 • **PREP TIME:** 10 MINUTES

The nutrients in kale play an important role in regulating inflammation and the stress response, as well as having antimicrobial properties, but kale tastes bitter due to an enzyme called glucosinolate. You can eliminate the bitterness by letting the kale sit in lemon juice, lime juice, or even vinegar for two minutes. If you are just starting to add kale to your diet and don't love the taste, toss a large batch of kale with lemon juice and store it in your refrigerator to use in salads or smoothies. But in this recipe, with sweet mango and spicy ginger, you won't notice the bitterness at all.

1 cup ice cubes

2 cups water

1 cup chopped peeled mango

2 cups baby kale

1 tablespoon minced fresh ginger

1 tablespoon agave syrup

1 medium banana, peeled

Put the ice, water, mango, kale, ginger, agave syrup, and banana in a blender. Blend until the mixture is smooth and creamy. Serve cold.

VARIATION TIP: If mangos are in season and particularly sweet, you can skip the agave.

PER SERVING: Calories: 143; Fat: 0.5g; Protein: 2g; Carbohydrates: 35g; Fiber: 4g; Sodium: 18mg; Iron: 1.5mg

Creamy Avocado Smoothie

SERVES 2 • **PREP TIME:** 5 MINUTES

If you have never made a smoothie with avocado before, definitely give this one a try. It's my version of creamy piña colada. Avocados are high in mono-unsaturated fat, which is considered a good fat because it helps lower your cholesterol. It's also full of vitamins, minerals, and fiber.

½ cup fresh or frozen pineapple chunks

1 ripe avocado

1 cup full-fat coconut milk

1 banana, peeled

1 cup ice cubes

2 tablespoons freshly squeezed lime juice

Put the pineapple, avocado, coconut milk, banana, ice, and lime juice in a blender. Blend until the mixture is smooth. Serve cold.

MAKE AHEAD TIP: This smoothie is best enjoyed immediately after serving, but you can also freeze it in an ice pop mold.

PER SERVING: Calories: 413; Fat: 35g; Protein: 4g; Carbohydrates: 29g; Fiber: 8g; Sodium: 21mg; Iron: 4.5mg

Pineapple-Coconut Smoothie

SERVES 2 • PREP TIME: 5 MINUTES

An enzyme in pineapple called bromelain has been shown to reduce inflammation, swelling, and even pain after surgery. This also makes it an excellent recovery food after strenuous exercise. Additionally, the abundance of vitamin C helps support immune function and growth. Try this smoothie as your post-workout snack.

1 cup water

½ cup ice cubes

1 cup full-fat coconut milk

2 cups fresh or frozen pineapple chunks

⅓ cup unsalted raw or roasted almonds

4 pitted dates

Put the water, ice, coconut milk, pineapple, almonds, and dates in a blender. Blend until the mixture is smooth and creamy. Serve immediately.

VARIATION TIP: If you can't find or don't like coconut milk, you can use 1 cup unsweetened almond milk and 2 tablespoons coconut oil.

PER SERVING: Calories: 523; Fat: 36g; Protein: 9g; Carbohydrates: 49g; Fiber: 8.5g; Sodium: 16mg; Iron: 5.5mg

Mango Lassi Smoothie

Many people think mangos are high-sugar fruits, but the natural sugar content is similar to that of apples and pears. Mangos are also high in vitamin C, vitamin A, fiber, and folate—one of the B vitamins that are essential for making red blood cells to carry oxygen around your body. Low levels of folate can lead to fatigue and even anemia.

1½ cups water

½ cup ice cubes

1 cup fresh or frozen mango chunks

2 tablespoons raw or roasted unsalted almonds

2 pitted dates

½ teaspoon vanilla seeds (optional)

Put the water, ice, mango, almonds, dates, and vanilla seeds (if using) in a blender. Blend until the mixture is smooth and creamy. Serve immediately.

MAKE AHEAD TIP: This smoothie keeps well in the refrigerator for up to 3 days. It's also great frozen in an ice pop mold.

HEALTH TIP: Vanilla extract is considered an acidic food, but vanilla beans are considered alkaline. Look for dried vanilla beans or bean pods.

PER SERVING: Calories: 143; Fat: 4.5g; Protein: 3g; Carbohydrates: 24g; Fiber: 3.5g; Sodium: 1mg; Iron: 0.5mg

Banana-Tahini Smoothie

SERVES 2 • PREP TIME: 5 MINUTES

Valued for their potassium levels, bananas aid in cardiovascular health. Potassium also helps maintain water balance within the cells in the body and helps counteract certain effects of dietary sodium. The proper balance of sodium and potassium in the body helps maintain healthy blood pressure levels. With the addition of almond milk, tahini, and dates, this smoothie offers the nutrients you need to start your day off right.

1 cup ice cubes

1 cup unsweetened almond milk

1 medium banana, peeled

2½ tablespoons tahini

2 pitted Medjool dates

¼ teaspoon ground cinnamon

Put the ice, almond milk, banana, tahini, dates, and cinnamon in a blender. Blend until the mixture is smooth and creamy. Serve immediately.

VARIATION TIP: You can substitute 2 tablespoons agave syrup for the dates. Or you can skip the sweetener altogether and add another banana.

PER SERVING: Calories: 224; Fat: 12g; Protein: 5g; Carbohydrates: 28g; Fiber: 3.5g; Sodium: 100mg; Iron: 1.5mg

Strawberry-Coconut Smoothie

SERVES 2 • **PREP TIME:** 5 MINUTES

Strawberries are one of my favorite fruits, especially in the peak early summer months. When I was young, I would eat a large bowl of strawberries with a small bowl of granulated sugar for dipping. I can't offer the same to my children, knowing what I know now as a registered dietitian, but it certainly brings back fond memories. This strawberry smoothie is what I serve instead. It's naturally sweet, creamy, and tart all at the same time.

1½ cups hulled strawberries

¼ cup raw cashews

2 pitted Medjool dates

1 cup full-fat coconut milk

¼ teaspoon vanilla seeds (optional)

1 cup water

1 cup ice cubes

Put the strawberries, cashews, dates, coconut milk, vanilla seeds (if using), water, and ice in a blender. Blend until the mixture is smooth and creamy. Serve immediately.

VARIATION TIP: You can use 1 cup water and 2 tablespoons coconut oil instead of coconut milk.

MAKE AHEAD TIP: This smoothie will keep in an airtight container in the refrigerator for up to 24 hours.

PER SERVING: Calories: 377; Fat: 30g; Protein: 6g; Carbohydrates: 25g; Fiber: 5g; Sodium: 18mg; Iron: 5mg

Green Breakfast Smoothie

SERVES 2 • **PREP TIME:** 5 MINUTES

This breakfast smoothie packs so many nutrients in a single glass! It also comes together in about five minutes, so you have no excuse to skip break- fast. You can even drink it on the go when you don't have enough time for a sit-down meal. Make this ahead and keep frozen for up to one month for busy days. All you have to do is thaw it overnight and it will be ready for you in the morning.

1 cup ice cubes

2 cups unsweetened almond milk

1 cup chopped kale

1 cup coarsely chopped peeled zucchini

2½ tablespoons unsalted raw or roasted almonds

2 pitted Medjool dates

Put the ice, almond milk, kale, zucchini, almonds, and dates in a blender. Blend until the mixture is smooth. Serve immediately.

INGREDIENT TIP: Zucchini is a good way to add fiber and nutrients to smoothies. An easy way to use it is to cube raw zucchini and freeze it so you can toss in a handful when- ever you'd like.

PER SERVING: Calories: 158; Fat: 8.5g; Protein: 5g; Carbohydrates: 16g; Fiber: 3g; Sodium: 194mg; Iron: 2mg

Cucumber-Kiwi Smoothie

SERVES 2 • **PREP TIME:** 5 MINUTES

Which fruit do you reach for when you want an extra dose of vitamin C? Most people will think of citrus fruits like lemons or oranges. But kiwi actually contains double the vitamin C of a lemon. So load up on kiwi the next time you go grocery shopping. When paired with cucumber, which promotes hydration, this smoothie is a perfect breakfast or a great midday snack when you are feeling a bit under the weather or need an extra boost of energy.

1 cup coarsely chopped seedless cucumber

2 kiwis, peeled and coarsely chopped

1 cup coconut water

1 tablespoon freshly squeezed lemon juice

10 fresh mint leaves

1 cup ice cubes

Put the cucumber, kiwis, coconut water, lemon juice, mint, and ice in a blender. Blend for about 60 seconds or until the mixture is completely smooth. Serve immediately.

MAKE AHEAD TIP: This recipe can be made ahead without ice and kept in an airtight container in the refrigerator for up to 24 hours. Pour it over ice to serve.

PER SERVING: Calories: 74; Fat: 0.5g; Protein: 1g; Carbohydrates: 17g; Fiber: 2.5g; Sodium: 35mg; Iron: 0.5mg

Coconut-Melon Smoothie

SERVES 2 • PREP TIME: 5 MINUTES

Melons are packed with fat-soluble vitamins, including vitamin A and beta carotene, which are better absorbed in our bodies when consumed with fat. This smoothie pairs melon with coconut (which is high in healthy fats) so you can absorb all the anti-inflammatory antioxidants in the most delicious way. If you prefer a creamier, thicker texture, use full-fat coconut milk instead of coconut water.

1 cup ice cubes

1 cup coconut water

2 cups
cantaloupe cubes

1 tablespoon
agave syrup

Put the ice, coconut water, cantaloupe, and agave syrup in a blender. Blend until the mixture is smooth and creamy. Serve immediately.

VARIATION TIP: This recipe is also great with ½ cup freshly squeezed orange juice. If you are adding orange juice, skip the agave syrup.

PER SERVING: Calories: 108; Fat: 0.5g; Protein: 1g; Carbohydrates: 26g; Fiber: 1.5g; Sodium: 57mg; Iron: 0.5mg

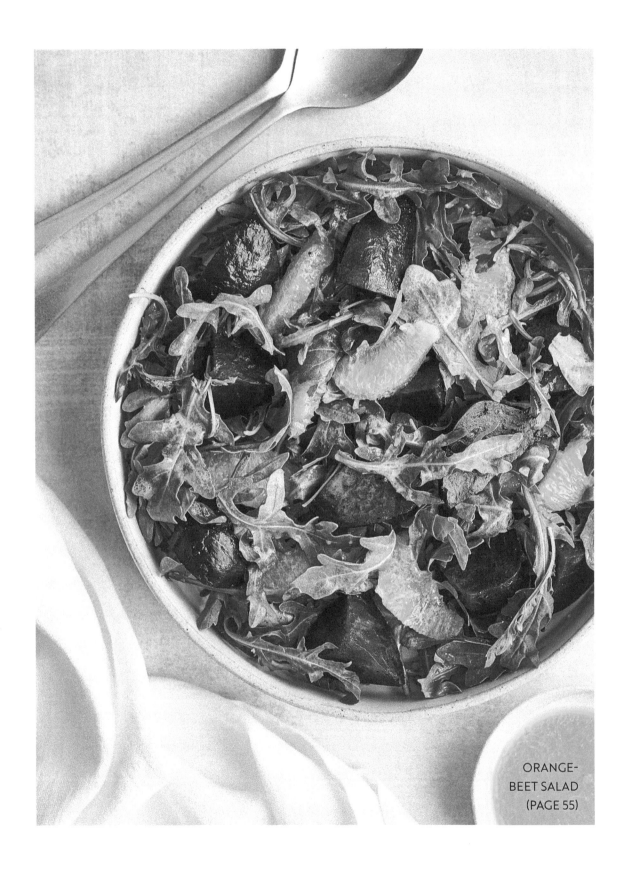

ORANGE-
BEET SALAD
(PAGE 55)

Salads and Soups

• • • • •

Crunchy Summer Salad

SERVES 2 • **PREP TIME:** 15 MINUTES

A meal without vegetables is not a complete meal, especially if you are following an alkaline diet. This salad is simple yet full of flavor and texture, making it the perfect accompaniment for any meal. The orange-mustard dressing is one of my favorites. It adds a sweet and tangy flavor and pairs well with all sorts of greens.

2 tablespoons extra-virgin olive oil

1 tablespoon orange juice

1 tablespoon Dijon mustard

⅛ teaspoon kosher salt

⅛ teaspoon freshly ground black pepper

4 cups romaine lettuce, cut into 2-inch strips

1 red bell pepper, cored and cut into ½-inch strips

1 cup seedless cucumber, cut into ½-inch-thick half moons

1. To make the dressing, in a large bowl, combine the olive oil, orange juice, mustard, salt, and pepper. Whisk together until it's well combined.
2. Add the lettuce, bell pepper, and cucumber. Toss to coat with the dressing.

MAKE AHEAD TIP: Romaine lettuce withstands dressing better than other leafy greens—which is why this salad can be made up to 2 hours in advance.

VARIATION TIP: If you like a more peppery flavor, you can use arugula instead of romaine lettuce.

PER SERVING: Calories: 172; Fat: 14g; Protein: 2g; Carbohydrates: 9g; Fiber: 3.5g; Sodium: 261mg; Iron: 1.5mg

Orange-Beet Salad

SERVES 4 • **PREP TIME:** 15 MINUTES

Beets are delicious, but it can be time-consuming to cook them from scratch. I often buy precooked, vacuum-packed beets that are ready to eat. The betalains in beets have anti-inflammatory properties that can help prevent and alleviate inflammation.

1 large orange

2 cups cubed (2-inch) peeled cooked beets

4 cups arugula

3 tablespoons extra-virgin olive oil

1 tablespoon Dijon mustard

1 tablespoon agave syrup

1. Over a bowl, peel and segment the orange by cutting between the membranes of each segment. Reserve all the juice from segmenting the orange.
2. To make the salad, in a large salad bowl, combine the beets, orange segments, and arugula.
3. To make the dressing, in a small bowl, combine the reserved orange juice, olive oil, mustard, and agave syrup until it's mixed well.
4. Pour the dressing over the salad and toss to coat. Serve immediately.

   VARIATION TIP: If you prefer tart over sweet, you can also use a grapefruit instead of an orange. You can also skip the arugula and add sliced cucumbers.

PER SERVING: Calories: 171; Fat: 10g; Protein: 2g; Carbohydrates: 18g; Fiber: 3g; Sodium: 360mg; Iron: 1.5mg

Fennel and Grapefruit Salad

SERVES 2 • **PREP TIME:** 15 MINUTES

Raw fennel has a licorice-like flavor and pairs well with citrus fruits like the grapefruit in this salad. Fennel is also a great source of fiber and has antibacterial properties. This salad also works well with oranges instead of grapefruit.

1 grapefruit

1 fennel bulb, cored and thinly sliced

2 cups arugula

1 ripe avocado, pitted, peeled, and cubed

3 tablespoons extra-virgin olive oil

1 tablespoon Dijon mustard

¼ teaspoon kosher salt

¼ teaspoon freshly ground black pepper

1. Over a bowl, peel the grapefruit, and segment by cutting between the membranes of each segment. Reserve all the juice from segmenting the grapefruit.
2. To make the salad, in a large salad bowl, combine the grapefruit segments, fennel, arugula, and avocado.
3. To make the dressing, in a small bowl, combine the grapefruit juice, olive oil, mustard, salt, and pepper. Mix well.
4. Pour the dressing over the salad and toss to coat. Serve chilled.

PER SERVING: Calories: 368; Fat: 31g; Protein: 3g; Carbohydrates: 22g; Fiber: 9.5g; Sodium: 386mg; Iron: 1.5mg

Cabbage Salad with Cashews

SERVES 2 • **PREP TIME:** 15 MINUTES

Kale may be the trendiest cruciferous vegetable right now, but cabbage is just as nutritious—and probably cheaper! Cabbage is packed with phytonutrients (nutrients found only in plants) and is high in fiber. Getting enough fiber daily can improve digestion and help lower blood sugar and cholesterol. Its vitamin C level is highest when raw, but there are benefits of cooking cabbage, too. Cooking unleashes an organic compound called indole that can fight off precancerous cells.

4 cups shredded red or green cabbage (or a mix of both)

⅓ cup coarsely chopped roasted unsalted cashews

2 tablespoons freshly squeezed lemon juice

3 tablespoons extra-virgin olive oil

1 tablespoon Dijon mustard

1 tablespoon agave syrup

1. Put the cabbage and cashews in a large mixing bowl.
2. To make the dressing, in a small bowl, combine the lemon juice, olive oil, mustard, and agave syrup until mixed well.
3. Pour the dressing over the cabbage mixture and toss to coat. Serve chilled.

VARIATION TIP: To mix things up, you can add other shredded vegetables, such as carrots, bell peppers, and cucumbers.

PER SERVING: Calories: 394; Fat: 31g; Protein: 5g; Carbohydrates: 27g; Fiber: 3.5g; Sodium: 222mg; Iron: 3.5mg

Tomato Carpaccio

Traditionally, carpaccio is a dish of meat or fish, thinly sliced or pounded thin and served raw. This tomato carpaccio is an adaptation, with tomatoes instead of the animal protein. It is probably one of my favorite summer recipes, and it's my go-to when I have friends over for dinner. It's so simple but really flavorful when prepared with sweet and juicy heirloom tomatoes. Ginger, lemon, and olive oil add a nice kick—and of course, lots of vitamins, minerals, and antioxidants.

4 large heirloom tomatoes, thinly sliced

1 scallion, trimmed and thinly sliced

1 tablespoon grated fresh ginger

1 tablespoon freshly squeezed lemon juice

3 tablespoons extra-virgin olive oil

1. On a large plate, spread out the tomato slices.
2. In a small mixing bowl, combine the scallion, ginger, lemon juice, and olive oil. Mix well.
3. Place about ¼ teaspoon of the dressing onto each slice of tomato. Serve at room temperature or chilled.

INGREDIENT TIP: If you don't feel comfortable slicing tomatoes very thin, you can use a mandoline or cut them into cubes and simply toss with the dressing.

PER SERVING: Calories: 251; Fat: 21g; Protein: 3g; Carbohydrates: 16g; Fiber: 4.5g; Sodium: 20mg; Iron: 1mg

Cauliflower Tabbouleh

SERVES 4 • PREP TIME: 20 MINUTES

Traditionally, tabbouleh is a salad made of finely chopped parsley, with tomatoes, mint, onion, and bulgur. If you like tabbouleh, you will love my adapted grain-free alkaline version of it. The cruciferous powerhouse cauliflower is high in vitamins C and B$_6$. These are water-soluble vitamins that get destroyed in the cooking process, so it's best to eat cauliflower raw. This tabbouleh recipe is one of my favorite ways to enjoy raw cauliflower because it has a great crunchy texture and includes other high-antioxidant ingredients such as parsley and mint.

1 head cauliflower, riced (about 3 to 4 cups)

⅓ cup freshly squeezed lemon juice

4 scallions, trimmed and finely chopped

1 cup finely chopped fresh parsley

½ cup finely chopped fresh mint leaves

3 tablespoons extra-virgin olive oil

¼ teaspoon kosher salt

¼ teaspoon freshly ground black pepper

In a large bowl, combine the cauliflower, lemon juice, scallions, parsley, mint, olive oil, salt, and pepper. Mix well. Serve chilled or at room temperature.

MAKE AHEAD TIP: This salad can be made in advance and refrigerated for up to 24 hours.

VARIATION TIP: Try adding pomegranate seeds or chopped cashews for different flavors and textures.

PER SERVING: Calories: 135; Fat: 10g; Protein: 3g; Carbohydrates: 8g; Fiber: 3.5g; Sodium: 107mg; Iron: 3mg

Warm Lentil Salad with Arugula

SERVES 4 • **PREP TIME:** 10 MINUTES • **COOK TIME:** 10 MINUTES

When following an alkaline diet, I highly recommend incorporating plant-based proteins such as lentils to ensure you're getting the nutrients you need. Lentils are an excellent source of both protein and fiber. Although they are not a complete protein, when combined with other plant-based foods, such as beans and rice, they can provide high-quality protein similar to chicken and beef. Lentils are also high in folate and polyphenols, which act as antioxidants.

3 tablespoons extra-virgin olive oil

1 large onion, thinly sliced

1 tablespoon fresh thyme leaves

1 cup cooked lentils, warm

3 cups arugula

Juice of ½ lemon

1. In a large skillet, heat the olive oil over medium-high heat. Add the onion and thyme. Cook, stirring occasionally, for 10 minutes, or until the onion is caramelized. Remove from the heat.
2. In a large salad bowl, combine the cooked onion, lentils, and arugula. Toss well.
3. Finish with a squeeze of lemon juice and serve warm.

MAKE AHEAD TIP: You can make this salad without the arugula and keep it in your refrigerator for up to 3 days. It's best to add the arugula when you're ready to serve, since it can wilt and get soggy quickly.

VARIATION TIP: You can skip the arugula if you prefer a simpler lentil salad.

PER SERVING: Calories: 171; Fat: 10g; Protein: 5g; Carbohydrates: 15g; Fiber: 5g; Sodium: 106mg; Iron: 3mg

Warm Asparagus Salad
with Tomatoes

SERVES 2 • **PREP TIME:** 5 MINUTES • **COOK TIME:** 20 MINUTES

Asparagus is one of the easiest and most versatile vegetables to cook. You can sauté, grill, or even bake it in the oven, as in this hands-off recipe. It doesn't require much seasoning, either. It is also a good source of folate, an important nutrient for healthy pregnancy and general cellular function and growth. It's high in insoluble fiber, which can help regulate bowel function.

1 bunch asparagus, trimmed and cut into 4-inch pieces

1 pint cherry tomatoes, halved

1 large shallot, thinly sliced

3 tablespoons extra-virgin olive oil

¼ teaspoon kosher salt

¼ teaspoon freshly ground black pepper

1. Preheat the oven to 400°F.
2. In a large baking dish, toss the asparagus, cherry tomatoes, shallot, olive oil, salt, and pepper to combine. Bake for 20 minutes.
3. Remove the dish from the oven and mix well to combine. Serve warm.

VARIATION TIP: This recipe is great with fish. After baking the vegetables for 20 minutes, remove the dish from the oven, add 1 pound halibut fillets, and gently toss to coat with the vegetables and sauce from the dish. Put everything back in the oven for about 15 minutes to cook the fish in the sauce.

PER SERVING: Calories: 245; Fat: 21g; Protein: 4g; Carbohydrates: 14g; Fiber: 5g; Sodium: 153mg; Iron: 3.5mg

Steamed Leeks with Mustard Vinaigrette

SERVES 2 • **PREP TIME:** 5 MINUTES • **COOK TIME:** 10 MINUTES

Most people use leeks to add flavor to another main ingredient, but leeks are the star of this recipe. They not only are anti-inflammatory but also are good sources of prebiotics, which are crucial for your gut health. We have both good and bad gut bacteria, and prebiotics act as fertilizer for the good gut bacteria, also known as probiotics.

1 large leek, cut into 3-inch strips and rinsed thoroughly

1 tablespoon Dijon mustard

2 tablespoons extra-virgin olive oil

Juice of ½ lemon

½ tablespoon agave syrup

⅛ teaspoon kosher salt

⅛ teaspoon freshly ground black pepper

1. Pour 1 to 2 inches of water and bring to a boil.
2. Place the leeks in the steamer basket and steam for about 5 minutes, or just until they're tender. Remove from the heat.
3. To make the dressing, in a small bowl, combine the mustard, olive oil, lemon juice, agave syrup, salt, and pepper. Mix well.
4. Place the steamed leeks on a serving plate and drizzle with the mustard dressing.

INGREDIENT TIP: Make sure to clean thoroughly between the layers of the leeks, since they can hide a lot of dirt.

PER SERVING: Calories: 172; Fat: 14g; Protein: 1g; Carbohydrates: 11g; Fiber: 1g; Sodium: 259mg; Iron: 1.5mg

Roasted Sunchokes with Rosemary

SERVES 2 • **PREP TIME:** 5 MINUTES • **COOK TIME:** 25 MINUTES

Sunchokes, also known as Jerusalem artichokes, are the tuberous roots of a sunflower plant. They're an excellent source of potassium and iron. When raw, they are crispy like an apple, but they turn soft and starchy when cooked. In this recipe, you'll roast the sunchokes to get them really crispy on the outside while still turning them soft on the inside. If you want to try one raw, you can thinly slice it and toss it in a salad such as the Crunchy Summer Salad (page 54).

8 ounces sunchokes, quartered

1 large shallot, sliced

1 tablespoon chopped fresh rosemary

3 tablespoons extra-virgin olive oil

1 tablespoon grated fresh ginger

1 teaspoon paprika

1. Preheat the oven to 400°F. Line a baking sheet with parchment paper.
2. In a large bowl, toss together the sunchokes, shallot, rosemary, olive oil, ginger, and paprika to coat.
3. Spread the sunchoke mixture out on the prepared baking sheet and roast for 25 minutes, or until they're tender inside and crispy outside. Remove from the oven.

PER SERVING: Calories: 258; Fat: 20g; Protein: 2g; Carbohydrates: 18g; Fiber: 2.5g; Sodium: 7mg; Iron: 3.5mg

Summer Gazpacho

SERVES 4 • PREP TIME: 20 MINUTES

Heirloom tomatoes are well loved for their flavor, but they are also packed with health benefits. Tomatoes contain lycopene, an immensely powerful antioxidant that prevents cell damage and atherosclerosis. This gazpacho is a delicious way to reap all the minerals, vitamins, and antioxidants of fresh tomatoes.

½ seedless cucumber, peeled

½ large red bell pepper, cored and coarsely chopped

2 pounds heirloom tomatoes, coarsely chopped

½ shallot, coarsely chopped

2 tablespoons sherry vinegar

1 teaspoon kosher salt

1. In a large bowl, combine the cucumber, bell pepper, tomatoes, shallot, vinegar, and salt. Let the mixture sit at room temperature for about 15 minutes.
2. Transfer the vegetable mixture, including all the liquid in the bowl, to a blender and blend until it's smooth. Serve cold.

MAKE AHEAD TIP: The vegetables can be cut and marinated overnight.

INGREDIENT TIP: If you can't find heirloom tomatoes or if they are not in season, go with beefsteak tomatoes or no-salt-added canned peeled tomatoes.

PER SERVING: Calories: 54; Fat: 0.5g; Protein: 2g; Carbohydrates: 11g; Fiber: 3.5g; Sodium: 292mg; Iron: 1mg

Simple Mushroom Broth

SERVES 4 • **PREP TIME:** 10 MINUTES • **COOK TIME:** 45 MINUTES

Mushrooms are the only plant-based natural source of vitamin D, which is crucial for maintaining bone and muscle health and energy level. When your body is low in vitamin D, you can experience fatigue, muscle weakness, and even depression. Plus, the rich flavor adds so much depth to this broth.

**2 tablespoons
extra-virgin olive oil**

1 medium onion, cut into cubes

½ leek, sliced and thoroughly rinsed

2 medium carrots, cut into cubes

1 tablespoon whole peppercorns

2 cups button mushrooms, halved

6 cups water

2 bay leaves

1. In a large pot, heat the olive oil over medium-high heat. Add the onion, leek, carrots, and peppercorns. Cook for about 5 minutes, or until the onion is translucent.
2. Add the mushrooms, water, and bay leaves. Reduce the heat to low and simmer for about 45 minutes. Remove from the heat.
3. Strain the solids through a strainer, reserving the liquid. Let it cool to room temperature before storing.

MAKE AHEAD TIP: The broth will last up to 3 days in the refrigerator and up to 1 month in the freezer.

PER SERVING: Calories: 74; Fat: 6.5g; Protein: 0g; Carbohydrates: 3g; Fiber: 0g; Sodium: 13mg; Iron: 0.5mg

Green Split Pea Soup

SERVES 4 • **PREP TIME:** 5 MINUTES, PLUS OVERNIGHT TO SOAK
COOK TIME: 30 MINUTES

This split pea soup is surprisingly good served warm or cold, and it makes for a great lunch, dinner, or even a snack. I like to add avocado slices and fresh oregano and thyme just before I serve it. Using a pressure cooker, you can cut the cooking time in half—no need for any other adjustments to the recipe.

2 tablespoons extra-virgin olive oil

½ onion, chopped into ½-inch pieces

2 celery stalks, cut into ½-inch pieces

1 cup green split peas, soaked overnight and drained

3 cups water, plus more as needed

1. In a large pot, heat the olive oil over medium-high heat. Add the onion and celery. Sauté for 3 minutes, or until the onion is translucent.
2. Add the green split peas and water. Bring to a boil. Cover the pot, and cook, stirring occasionally, for 25 minutes, or until the peas are very tender. Add more water if necessary. Remove from the heat.

MAKE AHEAD TIP: This is a good recipe to make in bulk and freeze in small containers so that you can enjoy it any time. It will keep in your freezer for up to 1 month.

PER SERVING: Calories: 242; Fat: 7.5g; Protein: 12g; Carbohydrates: 31g; Fiber: 12g; Sodium: 23mg; Iron: 2.5mg

Carrot-Ginger Soup

SERVES 4 • **PREP TIME:** 10 MINUTES • **COOK TIME:** 30 MINUTES

I like to have carrots in my refrigerator all the time. They're perfect to snack on raw and pair well with many meals. They're also a good source of beta carotene, the precursor for vitamin A, which leads to healthy cell function and plays a major role in vision. Ginger—the carrot's perfect pair—has been used for years to help with digestion, nausea, and inflammation.

1 tablespoon extra-virgin olive oil

1 cup diced onion

2 teaspoons grated fresh ginger

2 cups grated carrots

1 tablespoon apple cider vinegar

1½ cups water

1 (14-ounce) can full-fat coconut milk

1. In a large pot, heat the olive oil over medium-high heat. Add the onions and ginger. Sauté for about 5 minutes, or until the onion is translucent.
2. Add the carrots, apple cider vinegar, and water. Bring to a boil. Cook for about 20 minutes. Slowly add the coconut milk.
3. Transfer the mixture to a blender and blend until it's smooth.

MAKE AHEAD TIP: This soup can be kept refrigerated for up to 3 days or frozen for 1 month.

VARIATION TIP: You can use vegetable broth instead of water. Try Simple Mushroom Broth (page 65) for a rich flavor.

PER SERVING: Calories: 248; Fat: 24g; Protein: 2g; Carbohydrates: 8g; Fiber: 2.5g; Sodium: 51mg; Iron: 3.5mg

Leek and Potato Soup

SERVES 4 • **PREP TIME:** 5 MINUTES • **COOK TIME:** 30 MINUTES

Many people think white potatoes are bad and sweet potatoes are good, but each is very nutritious in its own way. White potatoes contain a type of starch called resistant starch. Because resistant starch is not fully broken down in your digestive system, it is a good source of nutrients for the good bacteria in your gut. Resistant starch can also help reduce insulin resistance and improve your blood sugar control.

2 tablespoons extra-virgin olive oil

1 small onion, chopped

1 large leek, sliced and rinsed thoroughly

5 Yukon Gold potatoes, peeled and cut into 2-inch cubes

5 cups water

2 teaspoons fresh thyme leaves

1 cup full-fat coconut milk

1. In a large pot, heat the olive oil over medium-high heat. Add the onion and leek. Sauté for about 5 minutes or until the onion is translucent.
2. Add the potatoes, water, and thyme. Bring to a boil. Cook for about 20 minutes or until the potatoes are tender. Add the coconut milk and mix well.
3. Remove the soup from the heat and transfer to a blender. Blend until it's smooth. Serve hot.

MAKE AHEAD TIP: This soup will keep in the refrigerator for up to 3 days or for 1 month in the freezer.

INGREDIENT TIP: You can use alkaline vegetable broth (try Simple Mushroom Broth, page 65) instead of water. You can also skip the coconut milk altogether.

PER SERVING: Calories: 318; Fat: 19g; Protein: 4g; Carbohydrates: 38g; Fiber: 2.5g; Sodium: 19mg; Iron: 5mg

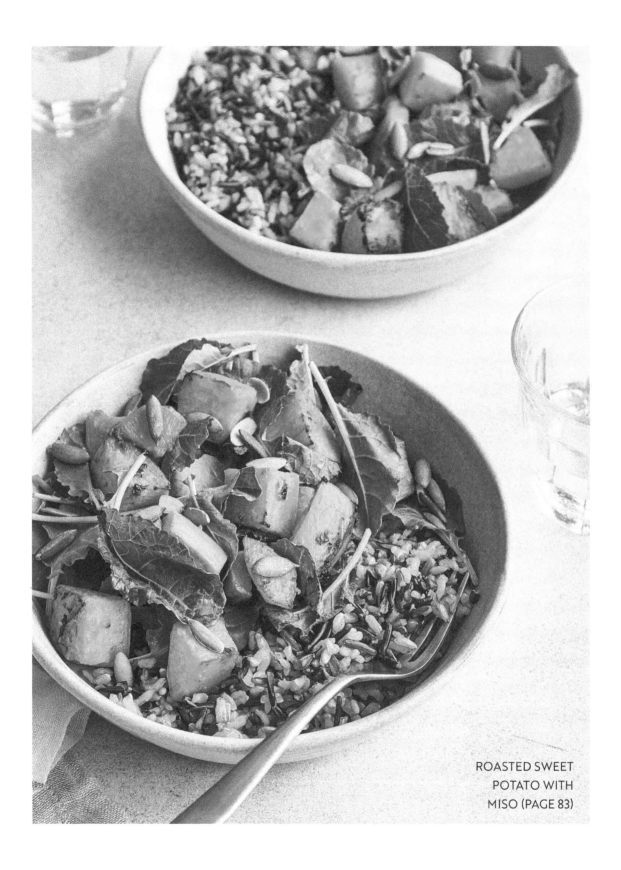

ROASTED SWEET
POTATO WITH
MISO (PAGE 83)

Entrées

• • • • •

Edamame and Cabbage Salad

SERVES 4 • **PREP TIME:** 5 MINUTES

Edamame (soybeans) are not only delicious but also high in protein and fiber. I usually make this recipe with frozen or vacuum-packed shelled edamame, because it takes very little time to make. It's great as a midday or late-night snack or as a full meal.

1 cup shelled edamame beans, cooked and drained

2 cups shredded green or red cabbage (or a mix of both)

2 tablespoons extra-virgin olive oil

1 tablespoon agave syrup

1 tablespoon apple cider vinegar

⅓ cup chopped fresh cilantro

⅛ teaspoon kosher salt

⅛ teaspoon freshly ground black pepper

In a large mixing bowl, combine the edamame, cabbage, olive oil, agave syrup, vinegar, cilantro, salt, and pepper.

MAKE AHEAD TIP: This salad can be prepared in advance and kept in the refrigerator for up to 2 days.

VARIATION TIP: You can add hemp seeds or chopped roasted cashews for extra crunchy and nutty flavor. And for a bit of heat, add ½ teaspoon hot paprika.

PER SERVING: Calories: 134; Fat: 8.5g; Protein: 5g; Carbohydrates: 10g; Fiber: 4g; Sodium: 50mg; Iron: 1.5mg

Potato and Sunchoke Salad

SERVES 4 • **PREP TIME:** 10 MINUTES • **COOK TIME:** 15 MINUTES

I am a huge fan of sunchokes, not only for their nutritional value but also for their taste and versatility. This recipe is an alkaline version of one of my favorite potato salad recipes. The simple dairy-free pesto adds so much flavor to the dish. If you have the time, try it with the Quick Pickled Radishes (page 118).

2 Yukon Gold potatoes, peeled and cut into 1½-inch cubes

2 cups sunchokes, cut into 1½-inch pieces

4 cups water

1 tablespoon grated fresh ginger

½ cup fresh basil leaves

¼ cup roasted unsalted almonds

2½ tablespoons extra-virgin olive oil

¼ teaspoon kosher salt

¼ teaspoon freshly ground black pepper

1. In a large saucepan, combine the potatoes, sunchokes, and water. Bring to a boil. Cook for about 15 minutes. Remove from the heat. Drain and let them cool.
2. To make the basil pesto, put the ginger, basil, almonds, olive oil, salt, and pepper in a blender or mini food processor. Blend until the mixture resembles a green paste.
3. Transfer the cooked potatoes and sunchokes to a serving bowl and top with the basil pesto.

MAKE AHEAD TIP: The basil pesto can be prepared ahead and kept refrigerated for up to 4 days.

VARIATION TIP: You can add 1 jalapeño pepper if you want to make the pesto spicy.

PER SERVING: Calories: 233; Fat: 13g; Protein: 4g; Carbohydrates: 28g; Fiber: 2.5g; Sodium: 76mg; Iron: 4mg

Wild Rice with Snow Peas

SERVES 2 • PREP TIME: 15 MINUTES

Wild rice isn't actually rice; it's the seeds of a wetlands grass that's native to North America. Wild rice is higher in fiber and 30 percent lower in calories than brown rice. I love the crunchy and nutty flavor, and it works well in salads because it is not as glutinous as brown rice, so the grains don't stick together. This warm grain bowl is good on its own but also works well with your favorite protein.

1 cup cooked wild rice

1 cup snow peas, cut lengthwise into strips

1 scallion, thinly sliced

2 tablespoons extra-virgin olive oil

1 tablespoon Dijon mustard

1 tablespoon freshly squeezed lemon juice

In a large mixing bowl, mix together the wild rice, snow peas, scallion, olive oil, mustard, and lemon juice to combine. Serve warm or cold.

MAKE AHEAD TIP: This recipe keeps well in the refrigerator for up to 3 days.

PER SERVING: Calories: 231; Fat: 14g; Protein: 4g; Carbohydrates: 21g; Fiber: 2.5g; Sodium: 184mg; Iron: 1.5mg

Cabbage and Cashew Stir-Fry

SERVES 4 • **PREP TIME:** 5 MINUTES • **COOK TIME:** 15 MINUTES

I am a big fan of taking shortcuts by buying prewashed leafy greens and pre-chopped vegetables. This warm stir-fried cabbage can be prepared in a flash using bags of preshredded cabbage. There is nothing wrong with taking shortcuts like that, especially if it means you can fit more healthy meals into a busy lifestyle. Enjoy this cabbage stir-fry with grains, proteins, or just as-is.

2 tablespoons extra-virgin olive oil

1 red onion, thinly sliced

4 cups shredded red cabbage

2 cups chopped bok choy

⅓ cup unsalted roasted cashews

½ cup thinly sliced dried apricots

⅛ teaspoon kosher salt

⅛ teaspoon freshly ground black pepper

1. In a large skillet, heat the olive oil over medium-high heat. Add the onion and cook for about 5 minutes, or until it's translucent. Add the red cabbage and sauté for about 3 minutes. Add the bok choy and cashews, and cook for 5 minutes. Remove from the heat.
2. Add the dried apricots, salt, and pepper to finish. Serve warm or cold.

INGREDIENT TIP: If you don't have red onions, you can use shallots or white onions.

PER SERVING: Calories: 201; Fat: 12g; Protein: 4g; Carbohydrates: 22g; Fiber: 4g; Sodium: 81mg; Iron: 2mg

Fried "Rice" Bowls

SERVES 2 • **PREP TIME:** 5 MINUTES • **COOK TIME:** 15 MINUTES

I make fried "rice" at least once a week, especially toward the end of the week, when I gather up all the leftover roasted and fresh vegetables and make a quick meal out of them for my family. This recipe uses quinoa to add high-quality plant-based protein that provides all the essential amino acids that animal proteins do. (See page 25 for instructions on how to cook quinoa.)

2 tablespoons extra-virgin olive oil

1 medium shallot, finely chopped

½ tablespoon grated fresh ginger

1 cup chopped mushrooms

1 cup chopped broccoli florets

¼ teaspoon kosher salt

½ teaspoon freshly ground black pepper

1 cup cooked quinoa

1. In a large skillet, heat the olive oil over medium-high heat. Add the shallot and sauté for about 2 minutes. Add the ginger, mushrooms, and broccoli. Sauté for about 3 minutes. Season with the salt and pepper.
2. Add the cooked quinoa, and sauté for about 2 minutes. Remove from the heat. Serve warm.

MAKE AHEAD TIP: This dish can be made ahead and kept in the refrigerator for up to 3 days.

VARIATION TIP: Add your favorite vegetables for different variations on this dish. Try carrots, zucchini, and cabbage—or whatever you have in the refrigerator.

PER SERVING: Calories: 269; Fat: 15g; Protein: 7g; Carbohydrates: 27g; Fiber: 5g; Sodium: 166mg; Iron: 2mg

Lentil Pasta with Summer Vegetables

SERVES 2 • **PREP TIME:** 5 MINUTES • **COOK TIME:** 25 MINUTES

Nowadays, you can find 100 percent lentil pasta that you can include in your alkaline diet without having to eat acidic wheat-based pasta. How amazing is that! There are so many lentil pasta types out there. Always read the ingredient list, and choose brands that contain only lentils to avoid unnecessary gums and additives.

4 cups water

1 cup lentil pasta

3 tablespoons extra-virgin olive oil

1 large shallot, thinly sliced

2 medium yellow or green zucchini (or a mix of both), cut into ½-inch-thick half moons

1 pint cherry tomatoes, halved

⅓ cup loosely packed basil leaves, chopped

⅛ teaspoon kosher salt

⅛ teaspoon freshly ground black pepper

1. In a small saucepan, bring the water to boil over high heat. Cook the lentil pasta according to the box instructions and drain.
2. In a large skillet, heat the olive oil over medium-high heat. Add the shallot, and cook for 2 minutes, or until they're translucent. Add the zucchini and tomatoes. Cook for 5 to 7 minutes, or until the tomatoes are darker in color.
3. Add the cooked lentil pasta, basil, salt, and pepper. Stir gently to combine. Remove from the heat. Serve warm or cold.

VARIATION TIP: For extra flavor, I like to add 1 or 2 garlic cloves (acidic) when sautéing the shallots, but you can leave them out to keep this dish 100 percent alkaline.

PER SERVING: Calories: 404; Fat: 22g; Protein: 13g; Carbohydrates: 39g; Fiber: 7g; Sodium: 96mg; Iron: 3mg

Butternut Squash with Lentils

SERVES 2 • **PREP TIME:** 5 MINUTES • **COOK TIME:** 20 MINUTES

Butternut squash is an amazing source of vitamins A, C, and E, as well as minerals, antioxidants, and fiber. Incorporating winter squash into your diet is a great way to boost your intake of antioxidants to prevent damage to your cells, which helps prevent many diseases.

2 cups cubed (1-inch) peeled butternut squash

½ medium red onion, sliced ½ inch thick

2 tablespoons extra-virgin olive oil

¼ teaspoon kosher salt

¼ teaspoon freshly ground black pepper

½ cup cooked lentils

1 tablespoon fresh thyme leaves

Grated zest and juice of 1 lemon

1. Preheat the oven to 400°F. Line a baking sheet with parchment paper.
2. Put the butternut squash and onion on the prepared baking sheet, and toss with the olive oil, salt, and pepper. Bake for 20 minutes, or until the squash is fork tender.
3. Transfer the baked squash to a serving bowl, and add the cooked lentils, thyme, lemon zest, and lemon juice. Toss everything together and serve warm.

MAKE AHEAD TIP: This dish will keep in the refrigerator for up to 3 days.

PER SERVING: Calories: 252; Fat: 14g; Protein: 6g; Carbohydrates: 29g; Fiber: 7.5g; Sodium: 242mg; Iron: 4.5mg

Vegetable Tacos

SERVES 2 • PREP TIME: 10 MINUTES **• COOK TIME:** 10 MINUTES

You can certainly enjoy delicious tacos on the alkaline diet. For this recipe, jicama slices or lettuce leaves serve as the "tortilla," and mushrooms replace the meat. Oyster mushrooms especially have great meaty texture and are so delicious when lightly sautéed.

2 tablespoons extra-virgin olive oil

2 medium shallots, thinly sliced

1 cup sliced bell peppers, any color

2 cups sliced oyster mushrooms

⅛ teaspoon kosher salt

⅛ teaspoon freshly ground black pepper

1 ripe avocado, pitted, peeled, and sliced

1 cup fresh cilantro leaves

1. In a medium skillet, heat the oil over medium-high heat. Add the shallots and sauté for about 2 minutes. Add the bell peppers, oyster mushrooms, salt, and pepper. Sauté for 2 to 3 minutes. Remove from the heat.
2. Serve the vegetables on your preferred "tortilla," topped with the avocado slices and cilantro.

MAKE AHEAD TIP: You can make the taco filling in advance and keep it in the refrigerator for up to 2 days.

PER SERVING: Calories: 301; Fat: 24g; Protein: 5g; Carbohydrates: 20g; Fiber: 9g; Sodium: 98mg; Iron: 2mg

Loaded Sweet Potatoes

SERVES 2 • **PREP TIME:** 10 MINUTES • **COOK TIME:** 35 MINUTES

Who says roasted sweet potatoes can't be a main dish? I like to roast about four to six sweet potatoes early in the week and have them as a snack or incorporate them into my family meals. Because sweet potatoes are a starch, they can serve as your carbohydrate portion of the meal. This recipe uses mushrooms, kale, and leeks to load up the sweet potatoes, but mix it up with your favorite alkaline toppings.

2 sweet potatoes, halved lengthwise

2 tablespoons extra-virgin olive oil

½ cup thinly sliced leeks

1 cup mushrooms

2 cups baby kale

⅛ teaspoon kosher salt

⅛ teaspoon freshly ground black pepper

¼ cup chopped fresh cilantro

1. Preheat the oven to 425°F. Line a baking sheet with parchment paper.
2. Place the sweet potatoes, cut-side down, on the prepared baking sheet and roast for about 35 minutes. Remove from the oven. Place on a serving plate, cut-side up.
3. Meanwhile, in a large skillet, heat the olive oil over medium heat. Add the leeks, and sauté for about 5 minutes. Add the mushrooms, kale, salt, and pepper. Sauté for about 5 minutes, or until the mushrooms are browned and the kale is softened. Remove from the heat.
4. Using a fork, fluff the sweet potato flesh. Put one-quarter of the sautéed vegetables on top of each sweet potato half. Garnish with the cilantro.

MAKE AHEAD TIP: Bake the sweet potatoes in advance and warm them up in the microwave for 1 minute before topping with the vegetables.

VARIATION TIP: I like to add 1 tablespoon vegan pesto or hummus (acidic) to the vegetable mixture for a more intense flavor.

PER SERVING (2 SWEET POTATO HALVES): Calories: 261; Fat: 14g; Protein: 4g; Carbohydrates: 31g; Fiber: 5.5g; Sodium: 165mg; Iron: 2mg

Spaghetti Squash with Almond Pesto

SERVES 4 • **PREP TIME:** 5 MINUTES • **COOK TIME:** 45 MINUTES

Spaghetti squash is the best vegetable-based pasta if you plan on avoiding gluten altogether. There are so many vegetable-based noodle alternatives, such as zucchini noodles, butternut squash noodles, and beet noodles, but spaghetti squash noodles most resemble wheat pasta—without all the starch.

1 spaghetti squash, halved lengthwise and seeded

¼ cup plus 1 tablespoon extra-virgin olive oil

½ teaspoon kosher salt

1½ cups fresh basil leaves, plus a few extra for garnish

1 tablespoon freshly squeezed lemon juice

¼ cup almond butter

1. Preheat the oven to 400°F. Line a baking sheet with parchment paper.
2. Brush the inside of the butternut squash with ¼ cup of olive oil and sprinkle with the salt. Place the squash halves, cut-side down, on the prepared baking sheet, and bake for about 45 minutes.
3. While the squash is baking, prepare the pesto. Put the basil, lemon juice, and almond butter in a mini food processor or blender. Blend until the mixture resembles a chunky pesto.
4. Remove the baking sheet from the oven. Let the squash cool completely. Using a fork, scrape out the flesh of the squash. It should look like strings.
5. Put the spaghetti squash in a serving bowl and add 2 tablespoons of the pesto. Mix well to coat. Garnish with the basil leaves and drizzle with the remaining 1 tablespoon of olive oil to finish. Serve warm.

MAKE AHEAD TIP: If making the spaghetti squash and the pesto in advance, store them separately in the refrigerator for up to 3 days.

VARIATION TIP: If you can handle the slightly acidic garlic, add 1 clove to the pesto for more flavor.

PER SERVING: Calories: 339; Fat: 27g; Protein: 5g; Carbohydrates: 23g; Fiber: 6g; Sodium: 341mg; Iron: 2mg

Miso-Glazed Eggplants

SERVES 4 • **PREP TIME:** 5 MINUTES • **COOK TIME:** 20 MINUTES

One of my clients had a difficult time incorporating vegetables into her diet. When she mentioned that she loves miso-glazed cod, I shared this recipe with her. Eggplants can taste a bit bland on their own, but this salty miso glaze sauce adds so much flavor. Pair this dish with roasted sweet potatoes or serve it with quinoa mixed with fresh mint and scallions.

1 tablespoon white miso

1 tablespoon agave syrup

1 teaspoon grated fresh ginger

3 tablespoons extra-virgin olive oil

1 teaspoon apple cider vinegar

⅛ teaspoon freshly ground black pepper

4 Japanese eggplants

1. Preheat the oven to 425°F. Line a baking sheet with parchment paper.
2. To make the miso dressing, in a small bowl, combine the miso, agave syrup, ginger, olive oil, vinegar, and pepper. Mix well until it resembles a creamy dressing.
3. Cut the eggplants in half lengthwise and make diagonal slashes along the cut sides. Place the eggplants, cut-side up, on the prepared baking sheet. Using a spoon or a brush, coat the cut sides of the eggplant with the miso dressing.
4. Bake for 20 minutes, or until the eggplants are golden brown. Remove from the oven. Serve immediately.

MAKE AHEAD TIP: Although this recipe is best served warm, you can use the leftovers cold in your salad or in a grain bowl.

PER SERVING: Calories: 241; Fat: 10g; Protein: 5g; Carbohydrates: 31g; Fiber: 10g; Sodium: 165mg; Iron: 2mg

Roasted Sweet Potato with Miso

SERVES 4 • **PREP TIME:** 5 MINUTES • **COOK TIME:** 30 MINUTES

The salty flavor of miso paired with the sweetness of the sweet potato is perfection. The crunchy texture of kale and pumpkin seeds adds tons of flavor and mouthfeel to this simple yet satisfying dish. If you don't have sweet potatoes, try this with butternut squash instead. Add about ⅓ cup wild rice or quinoa to make this dish heartier. Serve with fresh cilantro and lime zest on top for extra flavor.

2 tablespoons extra-virgin olive oil

1 tablespoon miso

1 teaspoon agave syrup

1 sweet potato, cut into 1-inch cubes

2 cups baby kale

¼ cup toasted shelled pumpkin seeds

1. Preheat the oven to 425°F. Line a baking sheet with parchment paper.
2. In a large bowl, mix together the olive oil, miso, and agave syrup. Add the sweet potato, and toss. Put the sweet potato on the prepared baking sheet. Bake for 30 minutes, or until it's caramelized and fork tender. Remove from the oven.
3. In a large serving bowl, toss together the miso-roasted sweet potato, baby kale, and pumpkin seeds. Serve warm.

MAKE AHEAD TIP: The sweet potato can be roasted in advance. Warm it just before serving and toss it with the kale and pumpkin seeds.

PER SERVING: Calories: 150; Fat: 10g; Protein: 3g; Carbohydrates: 11g; Fiber: 2g; Sodium: 193mg; Iron: 1mg

Roasted Eggplants with Herbs

SERVES 2 • **PREP TIME:** 10 MINUTES • **COOK TIME:** 35 MINUTES

Many people feel intimidated by eggplants, but they are so easy to cook, especially if you roast them. I like to cut mine in small cubes and get it crispy outside and soft inside. Whenever I prepare this dish, only about half the eggplant makes it into the dish because all my family members love to snack on it as soon as it comes out of the oven. Roasted eggplants are so underrated!

2 medium eggplants, cut into 1-inch cubes

¼ cup extra-virgin olive oil

⅛ teaspoon kosher salt

⅛ teaspoon freshly ground black pepper

¼ cup chopped macadamia nuts

¼ cup chopped fresh mint leaves

¼ cup chopped fresh cilantro

Juice of ½ lemon

1. Preheat the oven to 425°F. Line a baking sheet with parchment paper.
2. Put the eggplants on the prepared baking sheet. Toss well with the olive oil, salt, and pepper to coat the eggplants. Bake for about 30 minutes, or until the eggplants are golden brown.
3. Remove the baking sheet from the oven and transfer the roasted eggplants to a large bowl. Add the macadamia nuts, mint, and cilantro. Toss everything together.
4. Serve immediately with a squeeze of lemon.

VARIATION TIP: If you like garlic, you can also roast garlic cloves (acidic) together with the eggplants, and add them in step 3.

PER SERVING: Calories: 489; Fat: 39g; Protein: 7g; Carbohydrates: 36g; Fiber: 17g; Sodium: 87mg; Iron: 3.5mg

Curried Cauliflower

When my clients ask me how they can reduce the inflammation in their bodies, I tell them to eat lots of plant-based foods and incorporate plenty of spices and herbs. Herbs are a potent form of antioxidant that fights harmful free radicals—not to mention all the flavor they add to food! This is my take on curried cauliflower, with lots of aromatic spices.

1 head cauliflower, cored and cut into 2-inch florets

1 red onion, cut into ¼-inch-thick slices

¼ cup extra-virgin olive oil

1½ teaspoons ground turmeric

1½ teaspoons ground ginger

1½ teaspoons ground cumin

¼ teaspoon kosher salt

¼ teaspoon freshly ground black pepper

1. Preheat the oven to 425°F. Line a baking sheet with parchment paper.
2. In a large bowl, toss together the cauliflower, onion, olive oil, turmeric, ginger, cumin, salt, and pepper to combine.
3. Spread the cauliflower mixture out in an even layer on the prepared baking sheet and bake for 20 minutes. Remove from the oven. Serve warm.

VARIATION TIP: Try adding toasted almonds or cashews to the finished dish to make this even more delicious.

PER SERVING: Calories: 174; Fat: 14g; Protein: 3g; Carbohydrates: 11g; Fiber: 4g; Sodium: 117mg; Iron: 1.5mg

Stuffed Bell Peppers

SERVES 4 • **PREP TIME:** 5 MINUTES • **COOK TIME:** 30 MINUTES

Stuffed peppers are a great way to use up leftovers. Add grains, roasted vegetables, nuts, seeds, and any dressing of your choice, and you can turn leftovers into a gourmet meal! I am using quinoa here, but mix it up with any alkaline grains. Try the tahini dressing on page 110 for a nutty and creamy take on this dish.

2 bell peppers, any color, cored and halved lengthwise

1 cup cooked quinoa

1 teaspoon herbes de Provence

1 tablespoon extra-virgin olive oil

½ cup chopped fresh cilantro

1 ripe avocado, pitted, peeled, and sliced

1. Preheat the oven to 400°F. Line a baking sheet with parchment paper. Cut 4 additional squares of parchment paper big enough to cover half a bell pepper.
2. Place the peppers, cut-side up, on the prepared baking sheet.
3. In a small bowl, combine the quinoa, herbes de Provence, olive oil, and cilantro. Mix well.
4. Scoop the quinoa mixture into the pepper halves and cover each half with a piece of parchment paper to keep the quinoa from drying out. Bake for 30 minutes. Remove the peppers from the oven, and top with the avocado.

VARIATION TIP: You can add ½ cup tomato sauce (acidic) and ¼ cup black beans (acidic) to the filling to make it hearty and moist.

PER SERVING: Calories: 154; Fat: 9.5g; Protein: 3g; Carbohydrates: 15g; Fiber: 4.5g; Sodium: 9mg; Iron: 1mg

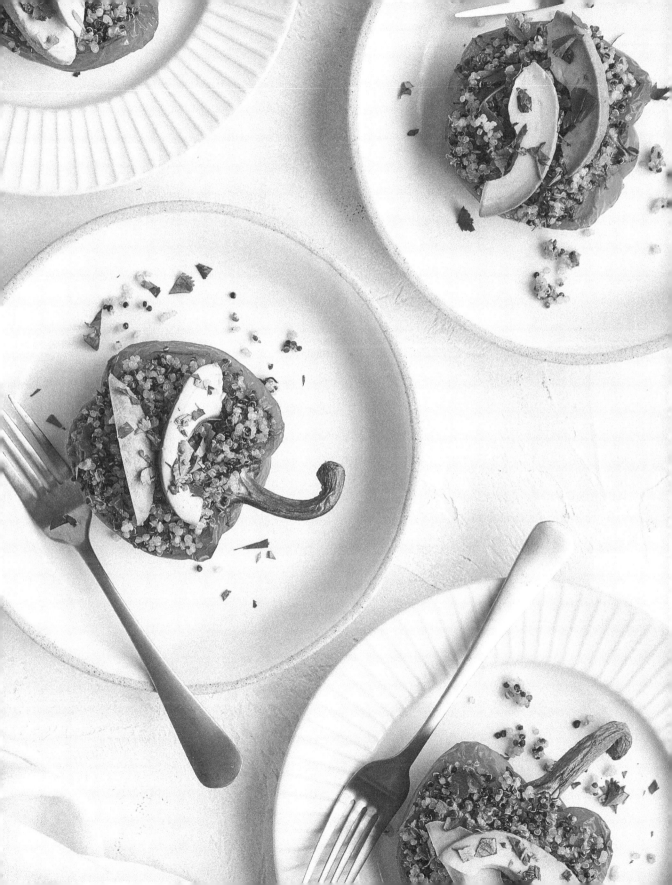

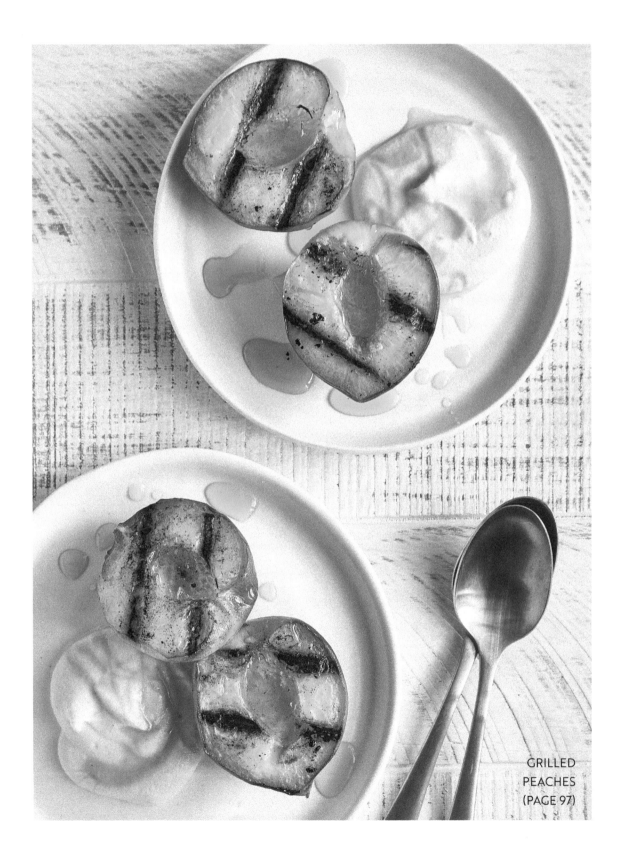

GRILLED
PEACHES
(PAGE 97)

Desserts

• • • • •

Strawberry Sorbet

MAKES 4 CUPS • **PREP TIME:** 5 MINUTES

Frozen fruits are great to use year-round. They are picked and flash-frozen at peak season, so they are fresh and nutritious. In fact, frozen berries have been found to be just as nutritious as fresh ones. This recipe also works well with raspberries and mint.

8 cups frozen strawberries

½ **cup water**

¼ **cup agave syrup**

Grated zest and juice of 1 Meyer lemon

1. Put the strawberries, water, agave syrup, lemon zest, and lemon juice in a blender. Blend to puree.
2. Serve immediately or freeze for up to 8 hours.

INGREDIENT TIP: A Meyer lemon is thought to be a cross between a lemon and a mandarin orange and is sweeter than a regular lemon. If you can't find one, you can also use half orange juice and half lemon juice for this recipe.

PER SERVING (½ CUP): Calories: 81; Fat: 0g; Protein: 1g; Carbohydrates: 19g; Fiber: 1g; Sodium: 4mg; Iron: 1mg

Coconut-Strawberry Ice Pops

MAKES 4 LARGE OR 8 SMALL • **PREP TIME:** 5 MINUTES, PLUS 5 HOURS TO FREEZE

These smoothie ice pops make for healthy and delicious treats—proving that great desserts don't always have to be loaded with sugar. I love to make these for my son year-round. If you don't have ice pop molds, small paper cups and wooden sticks work just as well. Simply peel off the paper when you're ready to eat them.

1½ cups frozen strawberries

1½ cups light or full-fat coconut milk

2 tablespoons agave syrup

2 tablespoons chia seeds

1. Put the strawberries, coconut milk, agave syrup, and chia seeds in a high-speed blender. Blend until the mixture is smooth.
2. Divide the mixture into ice pop molds (how many depends on the size of your molds) and freeze for at least 5 hours.

MAKE AHEAD TIP: These ice pops are great in the freezer for up to 1 week.

INGREDIENT TIP: You can use frozen or fresh strawberries. Fresh strawberries tend to add more sweetness, so if you are using them, leave out the agave.

PER SERVING (1 LARGE OR 2 SMALL POPS): Calories: 130; Fat: 6g; Protein: 1g; Carbohydrates: 19g; Fiber: 2.5g; Sodium: 31mg; Iron: 1mg

Lemonade-Ginger Ice Pops

MAKES 4 LARGE OR 8 SMALL   •   **PREP TIME:** 10 MINUTES, PLUS 5 HOURS TO FREEZE

Lemon not only is high in vitamin C but also can decrease the rate of kidney stone formation in some people. It is acidic in its natural state, but once metabolized in your body, it turns alkaline. So you can enjoy these refreshing lemonade ice pops on an alkaline diet. Meyer lemons work best, but you can use any lemons you can find.

Juice of 6 Meyer lemons (about 1½ cups)

Grated zest of 1 Meyer lemon

6 cups water

⅓ cup agave syrup

1 tablespoon grated fresh ginger

1. In a large bowl, combine the lemon juice, lemon zest, water, agave syrup, and ginger.
2. Pour the mixture into ice pop molds and freeze for at least 5 hours.

VARIATION TIP: You can leave out the ginger and substitute fresh mint, go with just lemon, or try lemon and strawberries.

PER SERVING (1 LARGE OR 2 SMALL POPS): Calories: 103; Fat: 0g; Protein: 0g; Carbohydrates: 29g; Fiber: 0.5g; Sodium: 0mg; Iron: 2mg

Alkaline Trail Mix

MAKES 4½ CUPS • PREP TIME: 5 MINUTES

When you don't have healthy ready-to-eat snacks around the house, that can lead to overeating at your next meal or snacking on processed foods. Make a large batch of this alkaline trail mix so everyone in the family can have a nutritious snack at any time of the day.

1 cup roasted unsalted walnuts

1 cup roasted unsalted cashews

1 cup roasted unsalted almonds

1 cup dried goji berries

½ cup toasted coconut chips (optional)

In an airtight container, combine the walnuts, cashews, almonds, goji berries, and coconut chips (if using).

MAKE AHEAD TIP: This recipe can be kept in the pantry in an airtight container for up to 2 weeks.

INGREDIENT TIP: Nuts are high in fat and can go rancid easily. It's best to keep them in the freezer if you want a longer shelf life.

PER SERVING (¼ CUP): Calories: 150; Fat: 12g; Protein: 4g; Carbohydrates: 9g; Fiber: 2g; Sodium: 16mg; Iron: 1mg

Stuffed Dates

SERVES 2 • **PREP TIME:** 5 MINUTES

My husband used to make these for me when I was pregnant with my son. Dates have been shown to promote easy labor and delivery. These also make for great pre- and post-workout snacks and are delicious when frozen!

6 pitted
Medjool dates

6 teaspoons
almond butter

12 raw almonds

1. Locate the cavity in each date left behind when the pit was removed.
2. Stuff each date with 1 teaspoon of almond butter and 2 raw almonds. Freeze or enjoy right away.

MAKE AHEAD TIP: These can be easily made ahead and kept in the refrigerator for up to 1 week. You can also freeze them for up to 1 month.

VARIATION TIP: I like to use almond butter and almonds for this recipe, but you can also make it with cashew butter and cashews.

PER SERVING: Calories: 260; Fat: 12g; Protein: 6g; Carbohydrates: 33g; Fiber: 5.5g; Sodium: 1mg; Iron: 1mg

Fresh Fig Tart

SERVES 8 • **PREP TIME:** 10 MINUTES

I used to make and bake tart shells from scratch for my fruit tarts. But after I started to make them with almonds and dates, as in this recipe, I never went back to my old recipe again. This fresh fruit tart requires no baking at all and is way more nutritious. Try using fresh berries instead of figs if you prefer.

1½ cups unsalted almonds

⅛ **teaspoon kosher salt**

2 cups pitted Medjool dates

4 cups fresh figs, quartered lengthwise

1. Put the almonds and salt in a food processor. Pulse until the mixture resembles coarse cornmeal. Add the dates and process until the mixture is uniform.
2. Press the mixture evenly into the bottom of a 9-inch springform pan.
3. Arrange the fresh figs over the top.

   MAKE AHEAD TIP: This tart can be refrigerated for up to 2 days.

PER SERVING: Calories: 252; Fat: 13g; Protein: 6g; Carbohydrates: 30g; Fiber: 6.5g; Sodium: 18mg; Iron: 1.5mg

Whipped Cashew Cream

MAKES 1 CUP • **PREP TIME:** 5 MINUTES, PLUS 6 HOURS TO SOAK

If you miss whipped cream, this easy recipe will be your new go-to. It's so creamy and flavorful that you will hardly believe it is completely plant based. Spoon this on the Strawberry-Rhubarb Compote (page 99), Baked Pears (page 100), Roasted Strawberries (page 101), or the Fresh Fig Tart (page 95). Top with chopped macadamia nuts for extra crunch.

1 cup raw cashews

½ cup water

1 tablespoon agave syrup

1. In a bowl, soak the cashews in enough water to cover for 2 to 6 hours. Drain.
2. Put the soaked cashews, water, and agave syrup in a high-speed blender. Blend for about 2 minutes, or until the mixture is smooth and stiff, like whipped cream.

MAKE AHEAD TIP: This cashew cream can be kept in the refrigerator for up to 24 hours.

VARIATION TIP: You can add about 1 teaspoon dried vanilla seeds, but keep in mind vanilla extract is not considered alkaline.

PER SERVING (2 TABLESPOONS): Calories: 87; Fat: 6g; Protein: 2g; Carbohydrates: 6g; Fiber: 0.5g; Sodium: 2mg; Iron: 1mg

Grilled Peaches

SERVES 4 • **PREP TIME:** 5 MINUTES • **COOK TIME:** 5 MINUTES

One of my son's favorite snacks, grilled peaches, is really simple to make even if you don't have a backyard grill. Simply use a cast-iron grill pan (or even a regular skillet) to get those nice grill marks. This is delicious drizzled with a little bit of honey or agave syrup or with a dollop of coconut yogurt, chopped almonds, or macadamia nuts on top.

1 teaspoon coconut oil

4 ripe summer peaches, halved lengthwise and pitted

2 tablespoons agave syrup or honey

1. Preheat your cast-iron grill pan (or a regular skillet) over medium heat. Coat the pan with the coconut oil.
2. Place the peaches on the pan, cut-side down, and cook for about 2 to 3 minutes.
3. Place the peaches, cut-side up, on a plate and drizzle with the agave syrup. Serve warm.

PER SERVING: Calories: 98; Fat: 1.5g; Protein: 1g; Carbohydrates: 22g; Fiber: 2g; Sodium: 0mg; Iron: 1mg

Grilled Pineapple Rings

SERVES 4 • **PREP TIME:** 10 MINUTES • **COOK TIME:** 10 MINUTES

This recipe was inspired by one of my favorite vegan restaurants. Sadly, it is no longer around, so I came up with this recipe to remember the flavors of their grilled pineapple dessert. It's sweet, crispy, and tart all at the same time. Simple yet delicious!

1 teaspoon coconut oil

4 fresh pineapple rings

1 tablespoon agave syrup

½ cup Whipped Cashew Cream (page 96) (optional)

½ cup coarsely chopped macadamia nuts

1. In a skillet or cast-iron grill pan, heat the coconut oil over medium-high heat.
2. Put the pineapple rings in the skillet and cook for 2 minutes on each side.
3. Transfer the cooked pineapple rings to a plate, and drizzle with the agave syrup, cashew cream (if using), and macadamia nuts.

MAKE AHEAD TIP: Pineapple rings can be cooked ahead and kept in the refrigerator for up to 2 days. Add the cashew cream, agave syrup, and nuts when ready to serve.

INGREDIENT TIP: You can use precut fresh pineapples or defrost frozen pineapple rings to save time.

PER SERVING: Calories: 164; Fat: 11g; Protein: 1g; Carbohydrates: 17g; Fiber: 2.5g; Sodium: 1mg; Iron: 1mg

Strawberry-Rhubarb Compote

SERVES 4 • **PREP TIME:** 5 MINUTES • **COOK TIME:** 15 MINUTES

I love making compote, especially in the summer. Seasonal fruits are so sweet and delicious that you don't need to add any sugar when cooking with them. You can store this compote in the refrigerator for up to 2 weeks, so make a big batch, and you'll have it ready when the craving hits for something sweet.

1 pound
strawberries, hulled

1 pound rhubarb, cut
into 2-inch pieces

2 tablespoons
agave syrup

1 tablespoon water

1. In a medium pot, combine the strawberries, rhubarb, agave syrup, and water. Cook, stirring occasionally, for about 15 minutes. Remove the mixture from the heat and set aside to cool completely.
2. When the mixture has cooled, transfer it to an airtight glass jar.

   VARIATION TIP: This compote is versatile and goes well with many sweets and toppings. I like to serve mine with ½ cup coconut yogurt and sprinkles of chopped almonds.

PER SERVING: Calories: 88; Fat: 0.5g; Protein: 2g; Carbohydrates: 21g; Fiber: 4g; Sodium: 5mg; Iron: 1.5mg

Baked Pears

SERVES 4 • **PREP TIME:** 5 MINUTES • **COOK TIME:** 25 MINUTES

Poached pears are such a simple and elegant dessert, and they're perfect for parties. But poached pears can take up to one hour to make, so I bake this modified version in the oven to save time. Top with whipped coconut cream or coconut yogurt and chopped macadamia nuts for a decadent treat.

1 teaspoon melted coconut oil

2 tablespoons agave syrup

½ teaspoon ground cinnamon

¼ teaspoon ground ginger

4 medium Bartlett pears, peeled, halved lengthwise, and cored

1. Preheat the oven to 350°F.
2. In a small bowl, combine the coconut oil, agave syrup, cinnamon, and ground ginger.
3. Place the pears, cut-side up, in a large baking dish, and evenly spread the coconut oil mixture over the tops. Flip the pears, cut-side down and bake for 20 minutes.
4. Flip the pears, cut-side up and bake for another 5 minutes. Remove from the oven.

MAKE AHEAD TIP: The pears can be made ahead and kept refrigerated for up to 3 days.

PER SERVING: Calories: 153; Fat: 1.5g; Protein: 1g; Carbohydrates: 35g; Fiber: 5.5g; Sodium: 2mg; Iron: 1mg

Roasted Strawberries

SERVES 4 • **PREP TIME:** 10 MINUTES • **COOK TIME:** 20 MINUTES

A cup of strawberries has more vitamin C than an orange! Similar to other berries, strawberries are high in fiber and antioxidants called polyphenols, which can lower chronic inflammation. Most importantly, nothing tastes better than sweet and juicy strawberries, especially on hot summer days! The roasting process brings out all the sweetness of strawberries.

1 pound
strawberries, hulled

½ cup chopped fresh
mint leaves

2 tablespoons freshly
squeezed lemon juice

1 teaspoon grated
lemon zest

¼ cup water

2 tablespoons
agave syrup

1. Preheat the oven to 425°F. Line a baking sheet with parchment paper.
2. On the prepared baking sheet, combine the strawberries, mint, lemon juice, lemon zest, water, and agave syrup. Mix well.
3. Roast for 20 minutes, mixing halfway through.
4. Let the berries cool completely before serving.

VARIATION TIP: This recipe is delicious on its own or topped with Whipped Cashew Cream (page 96) or coconut yogurt.

PER SERVING: Calories: 71; Fat: 0.5g; Protein: 1g; Carbohydrates: 17g; Fiber: 3g; Sodium: 4mg; Iron: 2.5mg

Coconut-Blueberry Bars

MAKES 12 BARS • **PREP TIME:** 10 MINUTES • **COOK TIME:** 40 MINUTES

When changing their eating habits, most people have a difficult time letting go of sweets. But when you have healthy dessert choices like this one that taste just as good, if not better, than the processed sweets you used to eat, you will feel so much more motivated to stick to your new routine.

1 tablespoon extra-virgin olive oil

2 ripe bananas, peeled and mashed

⅓ cup almond butter

¼ cup unsweetened almond milk

1½ cups unsweetened shredded coconut

½ cup fresh or frozen blueberries

1. Preheat the oven to 350°F. Grease a 9-inch square baking pan with the olive oil.
2. In a large bowl, combine the bananas, almond butter, almond milk, shredded coconut, and blueberries. Mix well.
3. Spread the mixture out in an even layer in the, prepared baking pan and bake for 40 minutes, or until the center is firm to the touch.
4. Let it cool completely before cutting into 12 bars.

MAKE AHEAD TIP: These bars are good in the refrigerator for up to 5 days.

VARIATION TIP: You can add about ½ cup seeds or nuts of your choice to the batter to make it heartier and increase the amount of omega 3 fatty acids. I like to add hemp seeds and chia seeds.

PER SERVING (1 BAR): Calories: 142; Fat: 11g; Protein: 2g; Carbohydrates: 9g; Fiber: 3.5g; Sodium: 4mg; Iron: 1mg

Almond Cookies

MAKES 40 COOKIES • **PREP TIME:** 10 MINUTES, PLUS 30 MINUTES TO CHILL
COOK TIME: 15 MINUTES

Yes, you can have cookies on an alkaline diet! These cookies are nutty, crumbly, and simple to make. I like to make a parfait with crumbled cookies, my Whipped Cashew Cream (page 96), and fresh berries, but these cookies are good as-is.

2½ cups almond flour

½ cup arrowroot flour

1 teaspoon
baking soda

2 teaspoons ground
cinnamon

½ cup agave syrup

¼ cup extra-virgin
olive oil or coconut oil

1. Preheat the oven to 350°F. Line 2 baking sheets with parchment paper.
2. To make the dough, in a large bowl, combine the almond flour, arrowroot flour, baking soda, cinnamon, and agave syrup. Mix well. Stir in the olive oil and gather the dough into a ball.
3. Divide the dough in half and roll each into an even log. Wrap with parchment paper. Let the logs of dough chill for about 30 minutes in the refrigerator.
4. Slice each log of chilled dough into 20 even rounds and place them on the prepared baking sheets.
5. Bake for 6 minutes, flip the cookies over, and bake for another 6 minutes.

   MAKE AHEAD TIP: If you love the recipe, you can make a large batch and keep it in your freezer for up to 1 month.

PER SERVING (2 COOKIES): Calories: 142; Fat: 7.5g; Protein: 4g; Carbohydrates: 15g; Fiber: 1g; Sodium: 63mg; Iron: 0.5mg

Watermelon Ice Pops

MAKES 4 LARGE OR 8 SMALL • **PREP TIME:** 5 MINUTES, PLUS 5 HOURS TO FREEZE

Ice pops are so easy to make and are perfect snacks for hot summer days. When you can find fresh and delicious fruit in season, take advantage, and make these ice pops. Swap in your favorite fruits if watermelon is not available. Throw into the blender whatever fruit is starting to wilt in the refrigerator.

4 cups coarsely chopped seedless watermelon

2 tablespoons agave syrup

1. Put the watermelon and agave syrup in a high-speed blender. Blend until smooth. Pour the mixture into ice pop molds.
2. Freeze for at least 5 hours before serving.

   VARIATION TIP: Add strawberries and mint for extra flavor.

PER SERVING (1 LARGE OR 2 SMALL POPS): Calories: 75; Fat: 0g; Protein: 1g; Carbohydrates: 19g; Fiber: 0.5g; Sodium: 1mg; Iron: 1mg

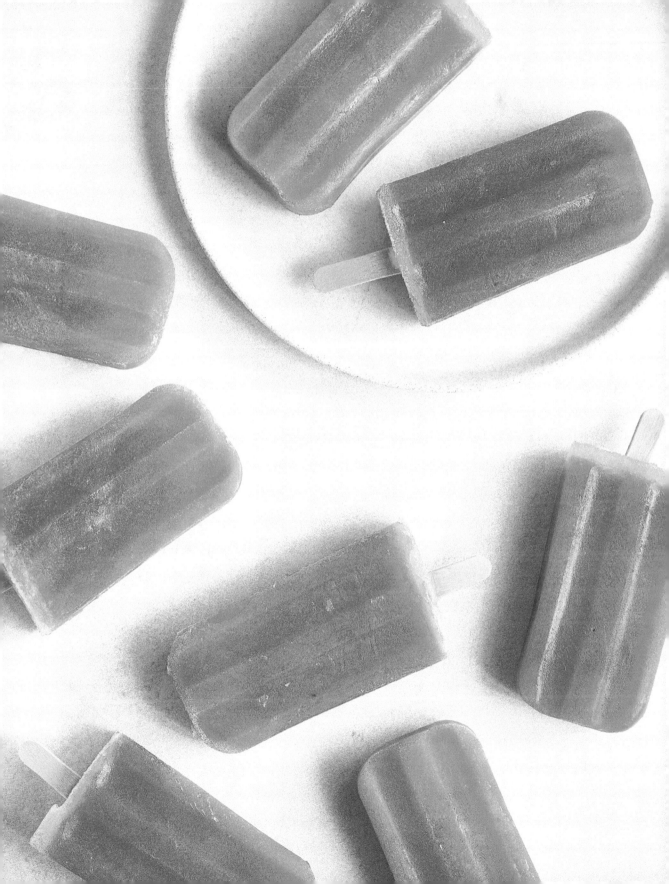

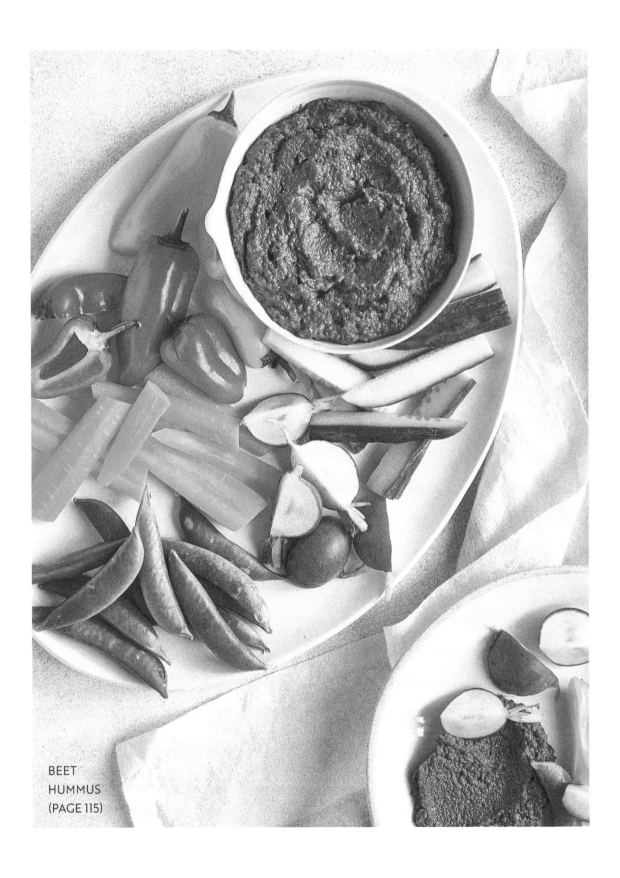

BEET
HUMMUS
(PAGE 115)

Staples and Snacks

• • • • •

Flax Egg

When you're following a mostly plant-based diet, cooking or baking without eggs can be a challenge. Flax seeds or chia seeds make for a great nutrient-dense and plant-based replacement for eggs. You can also just use these in a pinch when you've run out of eggs but still want to make pancakes!

2 tablespoons ground flaxseed

6 tablespoons warm water

In a small bowl, combine the ground flaxseed and warm water. Let it sit for about 5 minutes to thicken.

MAKE AHEAD TIP: You can make flax eggs ahead and keep them in the refrigerator for up to 1 month.

PER SERVING (1 FLAX EGG): Calories: 35; Fat: 2g; Protein: 1g; Carbohydrates: 2g; Fiber: 1.5g; Sodium: 0mg; Iron: 0.5mg

Cashew Cheese

MAKES 1½ CUPS • **6 SERVINGS** • **PREP TIME:** 5 MINUTES, PLUS 3 HOURS TO SOAK

Cashew cheese isn't just for people who follow an alkaline diet. It has a creamy texture and a nutty taste that is unique and addictive! This cashew cheese recipe pairs well with a variety of dishes, including salad, roasted vegetables, and Seed Crackers (page 119).

1 cup raw cashews

½ cup nutritional yeast

⅛ teaspoon kosher salt

1 teaspoon paprika

1 cup water

2 tablespoons freshly squeezed lemon juice

1. Put the cashews in a medium bowl with enough water to cover, and soak for 3 hours. Drain.
2. Put the cashews, nutritional yeast, salt, paprika, water, and lemon juice in a blender or food processor. Blend until the mixture is smooth.

MAKE AHEAD TIP: This cashew cheese can be made ahead and refrigerated for up to 3 days.

PER SERVING (¼ CUP): Calories: 135; Fat: 8g; Protein: 7g; Carbohydrates: 8g; Fiber: 2g; Sodium: 40mg; Iron: 1.5mg

Creamy Tahini Dressing

This tahini dressing goes well with any vegetables, but my favorite way to pair this dressing is with broccoli. It's also great on oatmeal, grain bowls, salad, and even on sliced apples with a dash of cinnamon. Make a big batch of this dressing on Sunday and keep it in the refrigerator to use on just about anything over the week.

½ cup tahini

¼ **cup water**

¼ **teaspoon kosher salt**

1 tablespoon freshly squeezed lemon juice

In a large bowl, mix together the tahini, water, salt, and lemon juice until creamy and smooth.

VARIATION TIP: You can add a minced garlic clove (acidic) for extra flavor.

PER SERVING (⅓ CUP): Calories: 357; Fat: 32g; Protein: 10g; Carbohydrates: 13g; Fiber: 3g; Sodium: 161mg; Iron: 2.5mg

Sesame-Miso Vinaigrette

MAKES ⅔ CUP • PREP TIME: 10 MINUTES

When a dressing is really good, it can transform even a boring salad into a special one. I love this sesame-miso dressing on steamed leeks. It's also great on any raw or roasted vegetables. You can also use the dressing to sauté vegetables. This calls for white miso for milder flavor. If you are using red miso, use half the amount.

¼ **cup extra-virgin olive oil**

2 tablespoons freshly squeezed lemon juice

2 tablespoons white miso

1 teaspoon apple cider vinegar

1 tablespoon sesame oil

½ teaspoon grated ginger

In a large bowl, combine the olive oil, lemon juice, miso, vinegar, sesame oil, and ginger. Mix well together until the vinaigrette is smooth and creamy.

MAKE AHEAD TIP: This recipe can be prepared ahead and refrigerated for up to 1 week.

VARIATION TIP: You can also add 1 tablespoon agave syrup for sweetness.

PER SERVING (⅓ CUP): Calories: 348; Fat: 34g; Protein: 2g; Carbohydrates: 9g; Fiber: 0g; Sodium: 662mg; Iron: 2.5mg

Creamy Avocado Dressing

MAKES 1½ CUPS • **PREP TIME:** 10 MINUTES

Unlike its other fruit cousins that are high in carbohydrates, avocados are uniquely high in fat. They also contain more potassium, which has been shown to lower blood pressure, than bananas. This creamy dressing is a delicious way to add tons of healthy fat and also fiber to any salad.

1 ripe avocado, pitted and peeled

¼ cup extra-virgin olive oil

¼ cup water

¼ cup fresh cilantro

¼ cup fresh basil leaves

Juice of 1 lime

¼ teaspoon kosher salt

¼ teaspoon freshly ground black pepper

Put the avocado, olive oil, water, cilantro, basil, lime juice, salt, and pepper in a high-speed blender. Blend until the mixture is smooth.

MAKE AHEAD TIP: This creamy dressing can keep refrigerated for up to 3 days.

VARIATION TIP: You can add 1 teaspoon grated garlic for extra flavor.

PER SERVING (2 TABLESPOONS): Calories: 60; Fat: 6g; Protein: 0g; Carbohydrates: 1g; Fiber: 1g; Sodium: 25mg; Iron: 0mg

Olive Spread

MAKES 1½ CUPS • PREP TIME: 10 MINUTES

Olives belong to the family of stone fruits and are related to cherries and pistachios. They are high in vitamin E, a powerful antioxidant that's great for your immune system. You can make this spread with any olives you like, but castelvetrano or kalamata olives work especially well. Paired with fresh parsley and lemon juice, this spread makes for a delicious, nutritious snack that is packed with antioxidants.

1 cup pitted and finely chopped castelvetrano or kalamata olives

¼ cup finely chopped fresh flat-leaf parsley

¼ cup extra-virgin olive oil

1 tablespoon freshly squeezed lemon juice

In a small mixing bowl, mix together the olives, parsley, olive oil, and lemon juice with a spoon to combine.

MAKE AHEAD TIP: This recipe can be made ahead and kept refrigerated for up to 2 weeks.

VARIATION TIP: You can add 1 teaspoon minced garlic or 2 tablespoons raisins for different flavor combinations.

PER SERVING (¼ CUP): Calories: 131; Fat: 14g; Protein: 0g; Carbohydrates: 0g; Fiber: 0g; Sodium: 602mg; Iron: 0mg

Kale Pesto

MAKES 1 CUP • 3 SERVINGS • PREP TIME: 10 MINUTES

It's hard to find store-bought pesto that does not contain acidic nuts and cheese. This recipe skips the nutritional yeast in favor of raw almonds to make the pesto extra nutty, and it's bright with kale and lemon juice. You can add a clove of garlic, if you tolerate it well, or replace half the kale with basil for a more traditional pesto flavor.

2 cups baby kale

½ cup extra-virgin olive oil

½ cup raw almonds

Juice of 1 lemon

¼ teaspoon kosher salt

Put the baby kale, olive oil, almonds, lemon juice, and salt in a food processor. Process until the mixture is smooth.

MAKE AHEAD TIP: This recipe can be made in advance and kept refrigerated for up to 1 week.

VARIATION TIP: You can skip the kale entirely and add all basil and a garlic clove for more traditional pesto flavor. I also love this recipe with cashews instead of almonds, since they add a creamy texture.

PER SERVING (⅓ CUP): Calories: 465; Fat: 48g; Protein: 6g; Carbohydrates: 7g; Fiber: 3.5g; Sodium: 106mg; Iron: 1.5mg

Beet Hummus

MAKES 2 CUPS • **PREP TIME:** 10 MINUTES

This hummus is perfect on salad, in grain bowls, and just as a dip with fresh, crunchy vegetables. I have tried variations using all sorts of vegetables, and they were all really delicious. My other favorites are parsley and sweet potatoes.

1 cup chopped
cooked beets

1 cup cooked shelled
edamame beans

2 tablespoons tahini

1 tablespoon grated
lemon zest

1 tablespoon freshly
squeezed lemon juice

¼ cup extra-virgin
olive oil

¼ teaspoon kosher salt

¼ teaspoon freshly
ground black pepper

Put the beets, edamame, tahini, lemon zest, lemon juice, olive oil, salt, and pepper in a high-speed blender. Blend until the mixture is creamy and smooth.

MAKE AHEAD TIP: This recipe can be made ahead and refrigerated for up to 5 days.

PER SERVING (⅓ CUP): Calories: 158; Fat: 13g; Protein: 5g; Carbohydrates: 7g; Fiber: 3g; Sodium: 152mg; Iron: 1mg

Babaganoush

MAKES 2 CUPS • **PREP TIME:** 5 MINUTES • **COOK TIME:** 40 MINUTES

This is my favorite Mediterranean starter. Traditionally, the eggplants in babaganoush are roasted directly on a fire, but you can also make this delicious spread in the oven. The tahini and lemon juice add extra depth of flavor. When I make this dish, it rarely lasts more than a day.

2 pounds eggplant

⅓ **cup extra-virgin olive oil, plus more for baking**

2 tablespoons freshly squeezed lemon juice

¼ cup tahini

2 tablespoons chopped fresh parsley

¼ teaspoon ground cumin

¼ **teaspoon kosher salt**

1. Preheat the oven to 450°F. Line a baking sheet with parchment paper.
2. Cut the eggplant in half lengthwise and brush the cut sides with olive oil. Place the eggplant, cut-side down, on the prepared baking sheet and bake for 40 minutes.
3. Remove the eggplant from the oven and let cool before scooping out the flesh with a spoon into a large bowl.
4. Add the olive oil, lemon juice, tahini, parsley, cumin, and salt. Mix well.

MAKE AHEAD TIP: This recipe can be made ahead and kept in the refrigerator for up to 3 days.

INGREDIENT TIP: You can rest the baked eggplant in a mesh strainer to drain out the liquid before adding other ingredients, but I personally find that the liquid adds so much flavor.

PER SERVING (⅓ CUP): Calories: 244; Fat: 22g; Protein: 3g; Carbohydrates: 11g; Fiber: 4.5g; Sodium: 54mg; Iron: 1mg

Pickled Ramps

MAKES 1 QUART • **PREP TIME:** 5 MINUTES • **COOK TIME:** 5 MINUTES

Ramps look like scallions but are mild in flavor. I usually either grill them and make pesto or pickle them. Unfortunately, ramp season is really short, so pickling them allows you to enjoy them a little longer. They are great on proteins, grains, or simple toast with avocados.

1½ cups distilled white vinegar

1 cup water

¼ cup agave syrup

3 pounds ramps, trimmed

1. In a medium saucepan, combine the vinegar, water, and agave syrup. Bring to boil. Cook, stirring occasionally, for about 3 minutes. Remove from the heat.
2. Put the ramps in a heatproof container and pour the hot liquid on them.
3. Let it cool completely, then cover with an airtight lid. Keep refrigerated.

MAKE AHEAD TIP: Pickled vegetables keep well in the refrigerator for up to 2 to 3 months.

VARIATION TIP: You can add fresh herbs or spices to this to make this even more flavorful.

PER SERVING (3 OR 4 RAMPS): Calories: 47; Fat: 0g; Protein: 2g; Carbohydrates: 11g; Fiber: 2.5g; Sodium: 16mg; Iron: 2mg

Quick Pickled Radishes

MAKES 1 QUART • **PREP TIME:** 10 MINUTES • **COOK TIME:** 5 MINUTES

Pickled vegetables can be a good source of probiotics and antioxidants, but they can also be high in sodium, and consuming too much salt can be bad for your health. Here is a salt-free recipe for quick-pickling vegetables, like radishes in this recipe, or red onions, carrots, or cauliflower florets. It takes no more than 30 minutes to make, and are a perfect side to any dish.

2 pounds small red radishes, thinly sliced

1½ cups distilled white vinegar

1 cup water

¼ cup agave syrup

1. Put the sliced radishes in a heatproof container.
2. In a medium saucepan, combine the vinegar, water, and agave syrup. Bring to boil. Cook, stirring occasionally, for about 3 minutes. Remove from the heat. Pour the boiling liquid on the radishes and submerge them in the liquid.
3. Let the mixture cool completely, then cover with an airtight lid. Keep refrigerated.

MAKE AHEAD TIP: Pickled vegetables keep well in the refrigerator for up to 2 to 3 months.

VARIATION TIP: You can add fresh herbs or spices, such as whole peppercorns and fresh dill, to this pickle to make it even more flavorful.

PER SERVING (¼ CUP): Calories: 9; Fat: 0g; Protein: 1g; Carbohydrates: 22g; Fiber: 3g; Sodium: 24mg; Iron: 0.5mg

Seed Crackers

SERVES 8 • **PREP TIME:** 15 MINUTES • **COOK TIME:** 45 MINUTES

Packed with fiber and protein, seeds are also a great source of omega 3 fatty acids, which have been shown to help alleviate mild to major depression. Our bodies don't make omega 3 fatty acids, so they are considered essential nutrients that must be eaten in our food. These crackers are also the perfect snack for new moms recovering from delivery or nursing and for anyone who needs an energy boost.

1 cup sunflower seeds

¾ cup pumpkin seeds

½ cup sesame seeds

½ cup chia seeds

¼ cup flax seeds

1½ cups water

¼ teaspoon kosher salt

1. Preheat the oven to 340°F. Line 2 baking sheets with parchment paper.
2. In a large bowl, combine the sunflower seeds, pumpkin seeds, sesame seeds, chia seeds, flax seeds, water, and salt. Let stand for about 15 minutes to thicken.
3. Divide the mixture evenly on the prepared baking sheets, and spread it into a layer about ¼ inch thick.
4. Bake, rotating the baking sheets halfway through, for 45 minutes, or until the mixture is crisp. Depending on the thickness, you may need to bake the mixture for another 5 minutes until it's golden brown. Remove from the oven.
5. Let it cool completely before breaking into small pieces.

   MAKE AHEAD TIP: This can be made in advance and kept in airtight containers for up to 1 week.

PER SERVING: Calories: 282; Fat: 23g; Protein: 12g; Carbohydrates: 11g; Fiber: 8g; Sodium: 56mg; Iron: 3.5mg

Baked Sweet Potato Fries

SERVES 6 • **PREP TIME:** 10 MINUTES • **COOK TIME:** 25 MINUTES

I grew up eating Japanese sweet potatoes. I like them fire-roasted, oven-baked, steamed, and even pan-fried with agave and sesame seeds. Japanese sweet potatoes are firmer and hold their shape nicely when you make fries with them. This is definitely one of my favorite recipes to make for my kids. The key to making crispy sweet potatoes in the oven is to use a rack.

3 medium sweet potatoes, cut into 1-inch matchsticks

3 tablespoons coconut oil, melted

1 tablespoon paprika

1 tablespoon dried oregano

⅛ **teaspoon kosher salt**

⅛ **teaspoon freshly ground black pepper**

1. Preheat the oven to 450°F. Line a baking sheet with parchment paper, and place a wire rack inside the baking sheet.
2. In a large bowl, combine the sweet potatoes, coconut oil, paprika, oregano, salt, and pepper.
3. Spread the sweet potatoes out on the rack. Bake for 25 minutes. Remove from the oven. Serve hot.

VARIATION TIP: You can use different spices, such as rosemary, cumin, or turmeric.

PER SERVING: Calories: 121; Fat: 7g; Protein: 1g; Carbohydrates: 14g; Fiber: 2.5g; Sodium: 60mg; Iron: 1mg

Baked Parsnip Fries

SERVES 6 • **PREP TIME:** 10 MINUTES • **COOK TIME:** 25 MINUTES

Move over, sweet potato fries! These parsnip fries are slightly crunchy outside and soft and chewy inside. If you generally like your fries that way, these are perfect for you. This recipe uses rosemary for seasoning, but you can use any seasonings you love, such as paprika and black pepper.

2 pounds parsnips, peeled and cut into 2-inch strips

3 tablespoons extra-virgin olive oil

½ tablespoon freshly ground black pepper

1 tablespoon finely chopped fresh rosemary leaves

½ teaspoon kosher salt

1. Preheat the oven to 425°F. Line a baking sheet with parchment paper.
2. Spread the parsnips out on the prepared baking sheet and toss with the olive oil, pepper, rosemary, and salt.
3. Bake for about 15 minutes, then toss the parsnips. Bake for another 10 minutes, or until the parsnips are golden brown. Remove from the oven. Serve immediately.

VARIATION TIP: This recipe also works great with carrots.

PER SERVING: Calories: 156; Fat: 7g; Protein: 1g; Carbohydrates: 23g; Fiber: 6.5g; Sodium: 106mg; Iron: 1mg

Sesame Snow Peas with Cashews

SERVES 4 • **PREP TIME:** 5 MINUTES • **COOK TIME:** 10 MINUTES

Snow peas are high in vitamin C, fiber, and protein, and they are so under-rated. Eat them raw with my Beet Hummus (page 115), thinly slice them and add to salads for a refreshing crunch or sauté lightly and season them with sesame oil, as in this recipe.

2 tablespoons extra-virgin olive oil

4 cups snow peas

2 tablespoons sesame oil

¼ teaspoon kosher salt

¼ teaspoon freshly ground black pepper

2 tablespoons sesame seeds

3 tablespoons chopped raw or roasted unsalted cashews

1. In a large skillet, heat the olive oil over medium-high heat. Add the snow peas and sauté for about 5 minutes.
2. Add the sesame oil, salt, and pepper. Sauté for another minute. Toss with the sesame seeds and cashews. Serve warm or cold.

MAKE AHEAD TIP: This recipe can be made ahead and kept refrigerated for up to 3 days.

PER SERVING: Calories: 217; Fat: 19g; Protein: 4g; Carbohydrates: 9g; Fiber: 2.5g; Sodium: 80mg; Iron: 2.5mg

Measurement Conversions

Volume Equivalents (Liquid)

US Standard	US Standard (ounces)	Metric (approximate)
2 tablespoons	1 fl. oz.	30 mL
¼ cup	2 fl. oz.	60 mL
½ cup	4 fl. oz.	120 mL
1 cup	8 fl. oz.	240 mL
1½ cups	12 fl. oz.	355 mL
2 cups or 1 pint	16 fl. oz.	475 mL
4 cups or 1 quart	32 fl. oz.	1 L
1 gallon	128 fl. oz.	4 L

Oven Temperatures

Fahrenheit (F)	Celsius (C) (approximate)
250°F	120°C
300°F	150°C
325°F	165°C
350°F	180°C
375°F	190°C
400°F	200°C
425°F	220°C
450°F	230°C

Volume Equivalents (Dry)

US Standard	Metric (approximate)
⅛ teaspoon	0.5 mL
¼ teaspoon	1 mL
½ teaspoon	2 mL
¾ teaspoon	4 mL
1 teaspoon	5 mL
1 tablespoon	15 mL
¼ cup	59 mL
⅓ cup	79 mL
½ cup	118 mL
⅔ cup	156 mL
¾ cup	177 mL
1 cup	235 mL
2 cups or 1 pint	475 mL
3 cups	700 mL
4 cups or 1 quart	1 L

Weight Equivalents

US Standard	Metric (approximate)
½ ounce	15 g
1 ounce	30 g
2 ounces	60 g
4 ounces	115 g
8 ounces	225 g
12 ounces	340 g
16 ounces or 1 pound	455 g

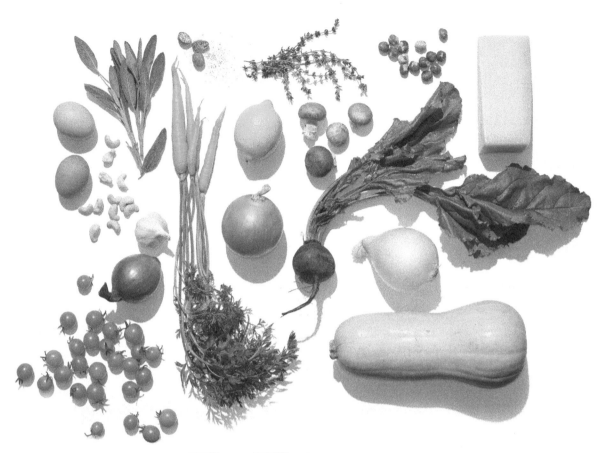

The Ultimate
Alkaline Food Guide

The Ultimate Alkaline Food Guide is a tool to support your health journey. Foods are ranked according to their levels of alkalinity or acidity. Any food within the alkaline range is fine to consume. When choosing foods in the acid range, aim for those that are low to medium in acidic value. That doesn't mean you can't enjoy a more highly acidic food every once in a while; just stick to the 80/20 rule.

This is a plant-driven guide, focusing on plenty of fruits and vegetables, including beans and legumes, and whole-grain foods (low to mildly acidic, but still very healthy for you). There is a wide variety of foods to choose from, plus flexibility per the spectrum of alkalinity and acidity provided. Be sure to limit highly processed foods, animal proteins, and dairy to special occasions.

Acid-Alkaline Ratings Charts

FOOD	ALKALINE			ACID		
	High	Medium	Low	Low	Medium	High

Alcoholic Beverages

FOOD	High	Medium	Low	Low	Medium	High
Beer					●	
Wine, red					●	

Vinegar and Oil

FOOD	High	Medium	Low	Low	Medium	High
Apple cider vinegar	●					
Avocado oil		●				
Balsamic vinegar			●			
Coconut oil		●				
Olive oil		●				

Beans and Legumes

FOOD	High	Medium	Low	Low	Medium	High
Adzuki beans				●		
Baked beans, vegetarian				●		
Black beans				●		

FOOD	ALKALINE			ACID		
	High	Medium	Low	Low	Medium	High

Beans and Legumes continued

FOOD	ALKALINE			ACID		
	High	Medium	Low	Low	Medium	High
Chickpeas				●		
Edamame			●			
Great northern beans				●		
Kidney beans				●		
Lentils	●					
Lima beans				●		
Navy beans				●		
Peanuts					●	
Peas, fresh green				●		
Peas, split green and yellow				●		
Pinto beans				●		
Snow peas			●			
Soybeans						●
String beans				●		
Tofu				●		

FOOD	ALKALINE			ACID		
	High	Medium	Low	Low	Medium	High

Beef/Pork

FOOD	High	Medium	Low	Low	Medium	High
Bacon						●
Frankfurters						●
Hamburgers						●
Steak (steaks, roasts, etc.)						●

Berries

FOOD	High	Medium	Low	Low	Medium	High
Blackberries	●					
Blueberries		●				
Cherries		●				
Raspberries	●					
Strawberries	●					

Beverages

FOOD	High	Medium	Low	Low	Medium	High
Apple juice, unsweetened			●			
Carrot juice				●		
Coconut milk, can or carton		●				

FOOD	ALKALINE			ACID		
	High	Medium	Low	Low	Medium	High

Beverages continued

FOOD	High	Medium	Low	Low	Medium	High
Coffee, regular					●	
Coffee, espresso						●
Cola						●
Grape juice		●				
Grapefruit juice	●					
Milk, 1% fat			●			
Milk, almond unsweetened		●				
Milk, nonfat			●			
Milk, rice					●	
Milk, soy			●			
Orange juice		●				
Tea, black			●			
Tea, green		●				
Tea, herbal		●				

FOOD	ALKALINE			ACID		
	High	Medium	Low	Low	Medium	High

Bread

FOOD	High	Medium	Low	Low	Medium	High
Bagel, plain						●
English muffins						●
Matzo, white flour						●
Pita, whole wheat flour					●	
Pumpernickel					●	
100% rye bread					●	
Tortillas, corn					●	
Tortillas, white flour						●
Whole wheat bread					●	

Dairy Products

FOOD	High	Medium	Low	Low	Medium	High
American cheese						●
Cheddar cheese						●
Cottage cheese					●	

	ALKALINE			ACID		
FOOD	High	Medium	Low	Low	Medium	High

Dairy Products continued

	High	Medium	Low	Low	Medium	High
Cream cheese					●	
Egg, white only				●		
Egg, whole				●		
Mozzarella cheese						●
Swiss cheese						●

Fish

	High	Medium	Low	Low	Medium	High
Bass					●	
Catfish					●	
Crab					●	
Flounder					●	
Grouper					●	
Salmon					●	
Shrimp						●
Tuna					●	

FOOD	ALKALINE			ACID		
	High	Medium	Low	Low	Medium	High

Flours

FOOD	High	Medium	Low	Low	Medium	High
Almond flour		●				
Amaranth flour			●			
Barley flour				●		
Buckwheat flour			●			
Millet flour			●			
Oat flour	●					
Rice flour, brown			●			
Wheat flour, white						●
Wheat flour, whole					●	

Grains

FOOD	High	Medium	Low	Low	Medium	High
Barley, whole grain					●	
Bulgur wheat					●	
Corn					●	
Cornmeal					●	

FOOD	ALKALINE			ACID		
	High	Medium	Low	Low	Medium	High

Grains continued

FOOD	High	Medium	Low	Low	Medium	High
Freekeh				●		
Kasha (buckwheat groats)				●		
Millet				●		
Oat bran					●	
Polenta					●	
Quinoa			●			
Rice, brown				●		
Rice, white					●	
Rice, wild			●			
Wheat, unrefined				●		

Fruits

FOOD	High	Medium	Low	Low	Medium	High
Apple		●				
Apricot		●				
Avocado		●				

FOOD	ALKALINE			ACID		
	High	Medium	Low	Low	Medium	High

Fruits continued

FOOD	High	Medium	Low	Low	Medium	High
Banana		●				
Cantaloupe	●					
Coconut			●			
Date				●		
Fig				●		
Grapefruit		●				
Grapes		●				
Kiwi fruit	●					
Lemon		●				
Mango	●					
Orange		●				
Papaya	●					
Peach		●				
Pineapple	●					
Plum				●		

FOOD	ALKALINE			ACID		
	High	Medium	Low	Low	Medium	High

Fruits continued

	High	Medium	Low	Low	Medium	High
Pomegranate					●	
Tomato				●		
Watermelon	●					

Herbs and Spices

	High	Medium	Low	Low	Medium	High
Basil		●				
Cilantro		●				
Cinnamon		●				
Cumin		●				
Curry			●			
Dill		●				
Ginger root	●					
Oregano		●				
Paprika	●					
Pepper, black		●				
Salt						●

FOOD	ALKALINE			ACID		
	High	Medium	Low	Low	Medium	High

Nut Butters

FOOD	High	Medium	Low	Low	Medium	High
Almond butter			●			
Cashew butter	●					
Peanut butter					●	

Nuts and Seeds

FOOD	High	Medium	Low	Low	Medium	High
Almonds			●			
Cashews	●					
Chia seeds			●			
Flaxseed			●			
Hazelnuts						●
Hemp seeds			●			
Macadamia nuts			●			
Peanuts					●	
Pecans					●	
Pistachio nuts					●	

FOOD	ALKALINE			ACID		
	High	Medium	Low	Low	Medium	High

Nuts and Seeds continued

Pumpkin seeds	●					
Sunflower seeds			●			

Pasta

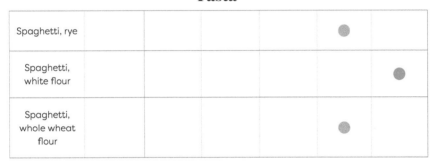

Spaghetti, rye					●	
Spaghetti, white flour						●
Spaghetti, whole wheat flour					●	

Poultry

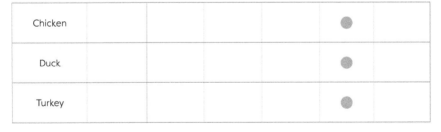

Chicken					●	
Duck					●	
Turkey					●	

FOOD	ALKALINE			ACID		
	High	Medium	Low	Low	Medium	High

Root Vegetables

FOOD	High	Medium	Low	Low	Medium	High
Beets		●				
Cassava		●				
Taro		●				
Yucca		●				

Sweeteners

FOOD	High	Medium	Low	Low	Medium	High
Agave nectar		●				
Artificial, aspartame					●	
Artificial, saccharin					●	
Corn syrup						●
Honey				●		
Maple syrup				●		
Molasses	●					
Stevia				●		
Sugar, brown						●
Sugar, white						●

FOOD	ALKALINE			ACID		
	High	Medium	Low	Low	Medium	High

Vegetables

FOOD	ALKALINE High	ALKALINE Medium	ALKALINE Low	ACID Low	ACID Medium	ACID High
Artichokes		●				
Asparagus	●					
Bell peppers		●				
Broccoli		●				
Brussels sprouts			●			
Cabbage		●				
Carrots, conventional				●		
Carrots, organic			●			
Cauliflower		●				
Celery		●				
Chard, Swiss				●		
Corn					●	
Cucumbers			●			
Eggplant		●				
Kale	●					

FOOD	ALKALINE			ACID		
	High	Medium	Low	Low	Medium	High

Vegetables continued

FOOD	High	Medium	Low	Low	Medium	High
Leeks		●				
Lettuce, arugula		●				
Lettuce, iceberg		●				
Lettuce, red leaf		●				
Lettuce, rocket		●				
Lettuce, romaine		●				
Mushrooms			●			
Mustard greens	●					
Okra		●				
Onions	●					
Parsnips	●					
Potato, white		●				
Potato, sweet	●					
Radishes	●					
Scallions		●				

FOOD	ALKALINE			ACID		
	High	Medium	Low	Low	Medium	High

Vegetables continued

FOOD	High	Medium	Low	Low	Medium	High
Spinach				●		
Squash, summer		●				
Squash, winter		●				
Yams	●					
Zucchini		●				

Water

FOOD	High	Medium	Low	Low	Medium	High
Bottled mineral, Evian		●				
Bottled mineral, Fiji		●				
Tap, chlorinated					●	

Miscellaneous

FOOD	High	Medium	Low	Low	Medium	High
Baking chocolate						●
Barbecue sauce					●	
Brownies						●
Butter				●		

FOOD	ALKALINE			ACID		
	High	Medium	Low	Low	Medium	High

Miscellaneous continued

FOOD	High	Medium	Low	Low	Medium	High
Burrito, with beef						●
Burrito, with chicken						●
Cheesecake						●
Croutons						●
Donuts						●
Horseradish	●					
Hummus				●		
Ketchup					●	
Mayonnaise				●		
Miso	●					
Mustard					●	
Pizza						●
Popcorn					●	
Potato chips						●
Tortilla chips						●

Resources

Imperfect Foods

ImperfectFoods.com
Imperfect Foods offers the convenience of having weekly fresh produce and groceries delivered to your home. Consumers are able to develop their own grocery lists and add their preferences. Then, each week they are sent a few selected items from Imperfect Foods, as well as the foods they picked online.

Local Harvest

LocalHarvest.org
Local Harvest helps you search for the closest farms and farmer's markets near you. To further develop community relationships with local farmers, there's also a directory of community supported agriculture (CSA) programs. CSAs enable consumers to buy seasonal products from local farmers. The consumer buys a membership or subscription and receives a box of fresh produce at regular intervals. This is a perfect way to support local farmers and receive healthy fresh produce.

National Farmers Market Directory

ams.USDA.gov/local-food-directories/farmersmarkets
With this directory from the USDA Agricultural Marketing Service, consumers can enter their zip codes to find the nearest vendor selling agricultural products. The directory shows locations, directions, times, and products offered at the farmers' markets near you.

Organic Consumers Association

OrganicConsumers.org
Organic Consumers Association (OCA) is a nonprofit organization that advocates for the interests of organic food and farming. OCA focuses on issues such as food safety, industrial agriculture, genetic engineering, sustainability, pesticides, and more.

References

Al-Kuran, O., L. Al-Mehaisen, H. Bawadi, S. Beitawi, and Z. Amarin. "The Effect of Late Pregnancy Consumption of Date Fruit on Labour and Delivery." *Journal of Obstetrics and Gynaecology* 31, no. 1 (2011): 29–31. doi.org/10.3109/01443615.2010.522267.

Anand, Preetha, Ajaikumar B. Kunnumakkara, Chitra Sundaram, Kuzhuvelil B. Harikumar, Sheeja T. Tharakan, Oiki S. Lai, Bokyung Sung, and Bharat B. Aggarwal. "Cancer Is a Preventable Disease That Requires Major Lifestyle Changes." *Pharmaceutical Research* 25 (2008): 2097–2116. doi.org/10.1007/s11095-008-9661-9.

Appleby, Paul N., Margaret Thorogood, Jim I. Mann, and Timothy J. A. Key. "The Oxford Vegetarian Study: An Overview." *The American Journal of Clinical Nutrition* 70, no. 3 (September 1999): 525s–531s. doi.org/10.1093/ajcn/70.3.525s.

Ceglia, Lisa, Susan S. Harris, Steven A. Abrams, Helen M. Rasmussen, Gerard E. Dallal, and Bess Dawson-Hughes. "Potassium Bicarbonate Attenuates the Urinary Nitrogen Excretion that Accompanies an Increase in Dietary Protein and May Promote Calcium Absorption." *The Journal of Clinical Endocrinology & Metabolism* 94, no. 2 (February 2009): 645–653. doi.org/10.1210/jc.2008-1796.

Dawson-Hughes, Bess, Susan S. Harris, and Lisa Ceglia. "Alkaline Diets Favor Lean Tissue Mass in Older Adults." *The American Journal of Clinical Nutrition* 87, no. 3 (March 2008): 662–665. doi.org/10.1093/ajcn/87.3.662.

Finkelstein, Eric A., Justin G. Trogdon, Joel W. Cohen, and William Dietz. "Annual Medical Spending Attributable to Obesity: Payer- and Service-Specific Estimates." *Health Affairs* 28, No. Supplement 1 (2009). doi.org/10.1377/hlthaff.28.5.w822.

Fraser, Gary E. "Associations between Diet and Cancer, Ischemic Heart Disease, and All-Cause Mortality in Non-Hispanic White California Seventh-Day Adventists." *The American Journal of Clinical Nutrition* 70, no. 3 (September 1999): 532s–538s. doi.org/10.1093/ajcn/70.3.532s.

Gans, Keri. "10 Most Searched Diets of 2020 on Google." *US News & World Report.* December 30, 2020. Accessed April 11, 2021. health.USNews.com/

health-news/blogs/eat-run/slideshows/10-most-searched
-diets-of-2020-on-google.

Harvard School of Public Health. "Simple Steps to Preventing Diabetes."
The Nutrition Source. Accessed April 13, 2021. hsph.harvard.edu
/nutritionsource/disease-prevention/diabetes-prevention
/preventing-diabetes-full-story.

Kelly, John R., Paul J. Kennedy, John F. Cryan, Timothy G. Dinan, Gerard
Clarke, and Niall P. Hyland. "Breaking Down the Barriers: The Microbiome, Intestinal Permeability, and Stress-Related Psychiatric Disorders."
Frontiers in Cellular Neuroscience 9 (October 14, 2015): 392.
doi.org/10.3389/fncel.2015.00392.

Kjeldsen-Kragh, J., C. F. Borchgrevink, E. Laerum, M. Haugen, M. Eek, O.
Frre. "Controlled Trial of Fasting and One-Year Vegetarian Diet in Rheu-
matoid Arthritis." *The Lancet* 338, no. 8772 (October 12, 1991): 899–902.
doi.org/10.1016/0140-6736(91)91770-u.

Knurick, Jessica R., Carol S. Johnston, Sarah J. Wherry, and Izayadeth
Aguayo. "Comparison of Correlates of Bone Mineral Density in Individuals
Adhering to Lacto-Ovo, Vegan, or Omnivore Diets: A Cross-Sectional
Investigation." *Nutrients* 7, no. 5 (2015): 3416-3426. doi.org/10.3390
/nu7053416.

Lanham-New, Susan A. "The Balance of Bone Health: Tipping the Scales in
Favor of Potassium-Rich, Bicarbonate-Rich Foods." *The Journal of Nutrition*
138, no. 1 (January 2008): 172S–177S. doi.org/10.1093/jn/138.1.172S.

Marques, Kelly K., Michael H. Renfroe, Patricia Bowling B. Brevard, Robert E.
Lee, and Janet W. Gloeckner. "Differences in Antioxidant Levels of Fresh,
Frozen, and Freeze-Dried Strawberries and Strawberry Jam."
International Journal of Food Sciences and Nutrition 61, no. 8 (2010):
759–769. doi.org/10.3109/09637481003796306.

McDougall, John, Bonnie Bruce, Gene Spiller, John Westerdahl, and Mary
McDougall. "Effects of a Very Low-Fat, Vegan Diet in Subjects with Rheu-
matoid Arthritis." *The Journal of Alternative and Complementary Medicine*
8, no. 1 (February 2002): 71–75. doi.org/10.1089/107555302753507195.

Monteiro, Carlos A. "Nutrition and Health. The Issue Is Not Food, Nor
Nutrients, So Much as Processing." *Public Health Nutrition* 12, no. 5
(May 2009), 729-731. doi.org/10.1017/S1368980009005291.

Remer, Thomas. "Influence of Nutrition on Acid-Base Balance—Metabolic Aspects." *European Journal of Nutrition* 40, (2001): 214–220. doi.org/10.1007/s394-001-8348-1.

Schieb, Linda J., Sophia A. Greer, Matthew D. Ritchey, Mary G. George, and Michele L. Casper. "Vital Signs: Avoidable Deaths from Heart Disease, Stroke, and Hypertensive Disease—United States, 2001–2010." *Morbidity and Mortality Weekly Report* 62, no. 35 (September 6, 2013): 721–727. CDC.gov/mmwr/preview/mmwrhtml/mm6235a4.htm.

Sutliffe, Jay T., Lori D. Wilson, Hendrik D. de Heer, Ray L. Foster, and Mary Jo Carnot. "C-Reactive Protein Response to a Vegan Lifestyle Intervention." *Complementary Therapies in Medicine* 23, no. 1 (February 2015): 32–37. doi.org/10.1016/j.ctim.2014.11.001.

Tonstad, Serena, Edward Nathan, Keiji Oda, and Gary E. Fraser. "Prevalence of Hyperthyroidism According to Type of Vegetarian Diet." *Public Health Nutrition* 18, no. 8 (September 29, 2014): 1482–1487. doi.org/10.1017/s1368980014002183.

Tonstad, Serena, Edward Nathan, Keiji Oda, and Gary E. Fraser. "Vegan Diets and Hyperthyroidism." *Nutrients* 5, no. 11 (2013): 4642–4652. doi.org/10.3390/nu5114642.

Tonstad, Serena, Terry Butler, Ru Yan, and Gary E. Fraser. "Type of Vegetarian Diet, Body Weight, and Prevalence of Type 2 Diabetes." *Diabetes Care* 32, no. 5 (May 2009): 791–796. doi.org/10.2337/dc08-1886.

Tucker, Katherine L., Marian T. Hannan, and Douglas K. Kiel. "The Acid-Base Hypothesis: Diet and Bone in the Framingham Osteoporosis Study." *European Journal of Nutrition* 40 (2001): 231–237. doi.org/10.1007/s394-001-8350-8.

Weaver, Connie M., Johanna Dwyer, Victor L. Fulgoni, III, Janet C. King, Gilbert A. Leveille, Ruth S. MacDonald, Jose Ordovas, and David Schnakenberg. "Processed Foods: Contributions to Nutrition." *The American Journal of Clinical Nutrition* 99, no. 6 (June 2014): 1525–1542. doi.org/10.3945/ajcn.114.089284.

Wolfson, Julia A., and Sara N. Bleich. "Is Cooking at Home Associated with Better Diet Quality or Weight-Loss Intention?" *Public Health Nutrition* 18, no. 8 (2015): 1397–1406. doi.org/10.1017/S1368980014001943.

Index